Mommy Dentists In Business

Mommy Dentists
In Business

Juggling Family and Life
While Running A Business

Dr. Grace Yum
Certified Pediatric Dentist

SILVER TORCH PRESS

SELF IMPROVMENT, BUSINESS DEVELOPMENT BOOKS AND MAGAZINES

Mommy Dentists In Business: Juggling Family and Life While
Running a Business © 2018 by Dr. Grace Yum

Printed in the United States of America.

ISBN: 978-1-942707-94-3
Library of Congress Control Number: 2018956941

MommyDentistsInBusiness@gmail.com
www.MommyDIBs.com

Published by Silver Torch Press
www.SilverTorchPress.com
Jill@SilverTorchPress.com

Table of Contents

Dedication

This book is dedicated to the following people:

my husband and kids,
Kent, Zoe, and Xander. I love you guys!

my family who love and support me.

my village of MDIBs all over the world.
We are the ultimate BossMoms!

Introduction

This book is meant to inspire all hard-working, hustling, busy moms that take care of their families and patients all while running their own businesses. I know that my own experience is different and my journey may be different, but I hope that you can take the basic principles and either see them in your own life or use them in the journey you are on. I wanted to write this book not just to share my own journey, but to encourage and support all Mommy Dentists who want to build their careers while building their own families.

Does anyone else feel like they are running around and making each day work? Yes, we have our fails and our successes but without both we can't appreciate the sweetness of success. I'm running to get out of the house and drop off at school, running to the practice, running to pick up. I just wish it was more cardiovascular! There are many of us Mommy Dentists in business and we need to support each other and build a bond so that no one feels isolated and alone. Dentistry can be isolating and it can be easy for us type-A personalities feel stressed out by our daily lives, but the beauty of our career is that we can make it work!

You're probably wondering why you should read this book and who I am. I am a first-generation Korean-American born and raised in Chicago, Illinois. My parents, from South Korea, immigrated to the US in the 1970's and have lived here ever since. My sister practices law in California. I have a loving husband who is extremely supportive of everything I do; he is my consigliere and partner in life. We have two wonderful children that are full of energy and love.

I grew up and lived in a north suburb of Chicago called Glenview until I attended college at Northwestern University. It wasn't until college that I started my career in dentistry and became a dental assistant. As a communications major and graduated with a bachelor of arts from the school of speech, I took a gap year and worked as an assistant for a consulting firm while working part time as a dental assistant. All four years, I worked for a pediatric and orthodontic office. The doctors had amazing lives and careers and encouraged me to pursue dentistry. I took the basic sciences just in case, but let me tell you, it was a struggle to get through them.

After a year of working in a consulting business, I was done and ready to go to dental school. It was so appealing to set my hours and be my own boss. I was accepted into the dental school in Maryland and lived in Baltimore for four years. All through dental school, I assisted in the orthodontic post-graduate clinic and faculty practice, even working as an assistant in private practice. Before I went to dental school, I really only had orthodontic experience and truly thought that I would go in that direction. As I had the opportunity to experience the pediatric department, I grew to love pediatric dentistry and wanted to pursue that road. I was required in my last year of school to do an externship and had the luxury of setting one up at Children's Memorial Hospital in Chicago for a week. It was an exciting time, and I loved every minute of it. I applied to the program and was very fortunate to be accepted at one of the top children's hospitals of Chicago. When I reflect on my life, I truly believe that it was the grace of God that opened doors to allow me to get where I needed to go. Certainly, it was not my own intelligence that got me this far.

Now that you have gotten to know a little about me, let's dig into the life of a Mommy Dentist in Business. I started a group on Facebook June 2017 and called it Mommy Dentists in Business. I wanted to create a group that had members in it that were like minded and shared the challenges of owning a business and raising children. Since then, I have met so many wonderful people with so much to share, that I felt compelled to invite them to share their stories alongside mine in this book. You will read my version of the chapter and then their story as well!

Chapter One
Get Help—Delegate

Evaluate your priorities and do what is best to make life do-able. This not only applies in your office but in your home as well. It took me a long time to figure out that I needed help and needed to surround myself with the right team. I came to the realization that sometimes it isn't worth the pressure of trying to perfectly execute everything by myself. Delegating is hard to do, but once you start to relinquish some control, you realize that you free up your time to do things that only you can do. If you can save your energy for your kids and your business, it will make you a better mom and boss. My husband travels for work, and often I am left alone during the week to act as a single mom. There is no way that I can get everything done by myself, so my husband and I decided that we would hire a team of people to help at home. Our children are little and need extra attention and care. Yes, they do go to preschool part time, but we also have two nannies and an assistant to run the house smoothly. That way when I come home from a long day, I don't have to worry about cooking, grocery shopping, dry cleaning, and managing contractors; instead, I get to come home and enjoy spending time with my kids. I couldn't live without my at-home team; in fact, they are just as valuable to me as my team at the office. They are in my home when I am not and are helping to raise my kids. It actually works out well because with multiple people present in my home, I don't feel the need to place security cameras in my house. I often joke around with my husband and tell him that my main nanny is my "wife," and that without her I would not be able to tend to my businesses and kids. He agrees that she takes care of all of us. The people that you hire to work inside your home are the most stressful hires because you are not physically present in the home to work with them. Most of the day, they are at your home without you. And if you have very young children, it can be more stressful because they cannot communicate to you what is going on in the home or if something is wrong. You might wonder if the nanny is engaging with your child or is she on her phone all day. Is the nanny truly watching my kids or is she running around doing whatever she wants? It truly is priceless when you can find people to work in your home that you completely trust, allowing you to fully engage at work without needing to check in constantly.

In addition to the importance of the team you hire at home in your daily life and routine, the team you choose at your dental office will make or break your day and stress levels. My team at the office operates and acts as though they are owners invested in the business. The office vision statement is visibly hung up in the break room, and we all help each other to work as effectively as possible. Again, without the right people, I have to work harder rather than smarter. My goal is to empower the team and let them work to the best of their abilities—to be the president of the business without micromanaging. It does not happen overnight, but it takes time to find the right people and situate them to work in the most fitting positions. I follow the motto, "Seat the right person in the right seat on the bus." I try to find the most appropriate people to do the job best suited for them and then train them to the best of their abilities. One of the best decisions I made was to hire an office manager. I wanted to reach the level where, as the CEO, I could just step into the office and focus on the work I know I need to do and not have to deal with things that can be handled by someone else. Initially, I was the one fixing time clocks and entering manual punches. I was the one who had to call the plumber if something was broken. I was the one who was reordering supplies. But once I started to delegate those responsibilities out to my office manager, I had more time to focus on dentistry, and that made me more productive at work and, therefore, more profitable.

Sometimes doctors feel nervous about handing over those responsibilities or even paying an assistant. I find that if you can see two new patients a day or do more dentistry, it pays for itself. As the business grows, the more the doctor's time needs to be protected; and the more unrelated tasks the doctor has to work on, the more opportunity cost is wasted. Surrounding yourself with the right people to work for you and offer you advice is so important in growing a successful dental business.

Introducing Dr. Stephanie Mapp

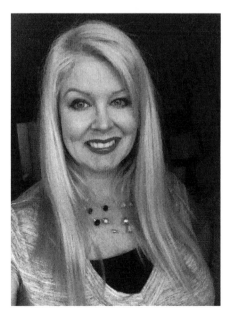

You worked your butt off to get great grades in undergrad to get into dental school. Then you worked your butt off in dental school and passed the boards to become a dentist. Now you are working your butt off to create a great practice where you can go out, conquer the world, be the diva of dentistry and stamp out tooth decay one restoration at a time. You are invincible, and you are going to have it all.

Yeah, your parents and friends and other family members have been supportive and helped you get to where you are, but *you* took all those tests, waxed all those crowns, set those denture teeth, and did all those required procedures like a one-woman army. The diva of dentistry will go forward and conquer practice ownership just like she conquered those requirements.

There's just one hitch. Although the diva of dentistry is a master of the handpiece, she has not had a ton of experience actually running a business. *What?! I have to run a business and do all this amazing dentistry?" the diva asks. The answer is yes. "No problem. I'll just take some online classes, go to some CE events, read a few books, and join a few Facebook groups to learn this stuff. Easy peasy.*

"It's not like it's biochemistry or embryology," the diva explains.

So the Diva goes and learns a lot about running an office. She's a fountain of knowledge of accounts receivable, profit and loss statements, insurance account aging reports. She's running her marketing campaign, doing her office Facebook account, paying her bills, ordering supplies, organizing the lab cases, sending her super organized QuickBooks account online to her accountant well before the tax deadline. She does all this in between hygiene exams, treatment plans, and giving anesthesia. She's a grade-A-type-A personality and she's got it all under control. Yes, I said *control*.

Did I mention that this diva of dentistry spends 10 to 12 hours a day at her office five or six days a week? She has no children and no social life. She watches Netflix and goes to the gym in her free couple of hours a day. She then eats a microwave Lean Cuisine, goes to bed, wakes up the next day, and does it all over again.

Wow. That sounds great, right?! Yeah, I didn't think so. But that's exactly the life you have as a practice owner unless you learn one important thing: delegate. You can't do it all. There aren't enough hours in the day.

One thing that is super difficult for us as tough, dynamic women dentists is to let go of some of the control we feel we must have to make our offices perfect. We spend most of our adult lives in control of our destiny through achieving our goals of becoming dentists and we want to apply that same control to the business. The problem is, a business requires a team; it is not a one-woman show.

"But I'm the diva of dentistry. I know the best way to do things so that they are perfect and up to my ideal standards. And if I let go of the reigns just a bit, these wild horses are going to go off running in all sorts of directions and never make it down the street for the big show. They won't do exactly what I want them to do," the diva protests. Sigh. Dearest Diva, don't you want to have a life and a family?

Isn't the reason you went through that torture of all-night-study sessions and lab work until 12am so that one day you could walk out of your practice at 5pm, get into your cute BMW with your Gucci key fob and your Louis Vuitton bag, pick Mini Diva up from ballet lessons, get home in time to throw on a cute little dress and go out for a nice family dinner? You will never live that fairy tale life if you don't learn this word: DELEGATE.

A quick google search yields a great definition of the verb delegate, "Entrust [a task or responsibility] to another person, typically one who is less senior than oneself." This is a very foreign word for many, many, many, many, many (did I say many?) women. I can't tell you how many very dear, smart, beautiful divas find this term to be very foreign. It is hard to let go. This is what I hear from many divas: "If I don't do this task, it won't be done properly." Or this one: "No one can do this task as well as I can." And then of course there's this one: "If I let someone else do this task and they get it wrong, I will have to eventually do it myself anyway, so I will just do it myself." Do these statements sound familiar?

I am here to tell you, Diva of Dentistry, that you need to get yourself a big sparkly magic wand and learn how to use it to become the director of your own orchestra. You need to be the maestro of your symphony. You need to wave that magic wand and move mountains by moving people to follow your direction in fulfilling your destiny of building your dental dynasty. Rome wasn't built in a day and it certainly wasn't built with Caesar schlepping those big ole rocks on his back to the location of the still-standing Coliseum. As a matter of fact, on a daily basis, you should be asking yourself, "Does this task require a DMD/DDS degree for it to be completed?" If the answer is no, you should not be doing it.

The toughest part of learning how to delegate is knowing how to begin. Understand that delegating is not an excuse to not know how to do something. In fact, the reason you are delegating the task, is that you know exactly how to do the task and you know it is something that does not take a degree to do. For example, you should understand how to run all of the necessary reports for your office within your practice management software. You should know how to file an insurance claim. You should know how to close out your accounts at the end of the day and send the credit card charges to the bank. But you should have protocols in place so that multiple people in your practice can do these things as well. You should know how to search how many outstanding insurance claims you have and how many days they have been outstanding and what percentage of your accounts receivable is from insurance versus patients who owe you out-of-pocket payments. Running the business really means you know how to run the business but you surround yourself with wonderful, capable people who can take care of many of the moving parts of your well-oiled machine while you supervise and take the very best care of your patients. Start making lists of what needs to be done on a daily, weekly, and monthly basis in your office. Get systems in place to teach your dynamic team how to do these things, and then get in there and run that handpiece and make some money, girlfriend, while the rest of your team takes care of the rest.

Once you have wrapped your noggin around the idea of delegating at your office, I want to give you one last diva challenge. Take a deep breath and think about all those little domestic tasks in your life that you don't have time to finish on a daily, weekly, and monthly basis. Go one step farther and think about the tasks that you do that may not be difficult but still take time away from your friends, family, or even your own free time; time that could be spent lounging on your bedroom chaise eating bon bons; or time you could spend getting a great mani-pedi. How about time you could be spending drinking margaritas on the beach in Cancun? We are talking the domestic chores of shopping, washing the dog, cooking dinner, changing the bed linens, vacuuming the car or the carpet, and driving Mini Diva to ballet lessons. Which of these tasks can be delegated? Too many divas believe they can and should do all of these things. Just because we know how to do them doesn't mean we should have to. Find good, capable people who can do these things for you. Why do it all? If you wanted to do all of these things, why did you bother going to dental school, instead of just finding a nice prince charming and staying home eight to nine hours a day to do them while he brings home the bacon? Becoming a diva of dentistry should help you get to a point where you can afford to delegate these things to someone who would love to have a great job. Men have wives to do these things; if you can't get a house husband to do them, pay for a wife of your very own. You may find different people to do some of these tasks. Ask your friends and neighbors for a trusted source. There are people out there.

11

One person can't and shouldn't have to do it all. You have proven yourself to be a formidable citizen of the world who carries the knowledge, the skills, and the compassion to be a successful dentist, business owner, wife, mother, sister, and friend to many. You can be accomplished and enjoy the fruits of your labor more completely by being more well-rested, less frazzled, and less scattered, by learning the art of delegation. Go forth, Divas of Dentistry, and rule the world.

Dr. Stephanie Mapp is a 1994 graduate of the University of Florida College of Dentistry. She started her college career following the footsteps of her father who was a psychologist. She chose dentistry as a career after becoming a patient at the dental college and realizing at that time dentistry was lacking female dentists. She obtained early admission to the dental college after only three years of undergraduate work. With over 20 years of dental experience, Dr. Mapp has worked in multiple types of dental settings including corporate group practices in North Florida as well as public health. She started her first practice more than 16 years ago and purchased a second location a few years later. She is a member of the American Dental Association, Florida Dental Association, Northeast District Dental Society and was a founding member of Clay Women in Business. In her free time, she loves to travel and spend time with her son and two dogs in her home outside Jacksonville, Florida.

To connect with Dr. Mapp, please contact her at DrMapp@hotmail.com.

Chapter Two

I Can Practice Dentistry
in my Sleep

Before delving into practice ownership, master your dentistry. Running a business and being a dentist are two totally different things. If you don't have the expertise in either field, things can get very stressful. You have to put in your time and effort. I hate to say it, but Rome wasn't built in a day. It takes a lot of hard work to get where you want to go. Nothing in life that is worthwhile comes easily. At the age of 19, while still attending college, I worked as an assistant. When I finally decided to start my first practice from scratch, I had been working as an associate for other dentists for five years. I had the opportunity to work in a myriad of offices, typically orthodontics and some pediatrics, before going to dental school. Eventually, I realized the owners of those practices taught me not only about dentistry and patients, but really so much more about the business aspects of being a medical professional than I had expected. I had worked my way up from sweeping floors, answering phone calls, and talking to insurance companies, to having my own chair and my own column—a huge accomplishment back then. All those experiences, no matter how brief, helped me to understand the inner workings of a private practice. By the time I attended dental school and progressed to becoming a full-fledged dentist, I already had under my belt in-depth experiences of how a practice operates. It was dentistry that I had to master. When I finally finished dental school, I decided to pursue pediatric dentistry and moved on to specialize in another two-year program. During my residency, I began to work as an associate where I gained essential insight into what a dentistry business entails. Even though there were long commutes and six-day work weeks, I built up speed, learned to sell treatment plans, and developed more confidence in communicating with patients and parents.

The point is that you have to put in your time to become a practitioner with experience. There is so much to learn outside of school that you can only learn on the job. One patient can see three different dentists and have more than one treatment plan. It is much harder to manage a practice and run a business if you don't know how to treat properly and efficiently. There is something to be said about hands-on experience that builds your confidence, but also changes your craft. Let's face it, dentistry is a trade and like all trades, it takes time to master it. One of my favorite movies is *Jiro dreams of Sushi*; sushi chefs spend their entire lives mastering their skill sets. One chef made tamago and another, seaweed, for 10 years before moving on to another skill. The point is that it takes time to master your craft. I firmly believe that with experience, you build your intuition and sense of things. Sometimes you don't know what or why or how to explain things; you just make decisions and sometimes those decisions are not based on dental school textbooks but rather on your experience. Take the time to learn dentistry and master it and be the best you can be.

Not only do you have to be able to practice your clinical skill sets, you need to develop communications skills. How do you talk and present to your patients? What can you do differently to obtain 100% treatment consent and acceptance? How do you know that the patient is fully understanding what it is you are talking about? I'd say that 80% of how a patient feels about his or her dentist is in how one presents himself or herself and develops a relationship with the patient. I'm not saying that you have to win over every single person that walks in the door, but there are patients who don't connect for whatever reason and they move on. Other patients will connect right away and feel at ease with their provider, but the more you connect with patients and the more you explain to them about their health and the condition of their health, the more they are going to trust you and move forward with their treatment. These are skills that aren't built overnight and are not taught in school. Developing people skills is just as important as having excellent clinical skills.

Introducing Dr. Nada Albatish

We all know the hardest part of dentistry. It's when you walk into first-year anatomy's human cadaver lab; some people faint, some cry, and some vomit into the nearest wastebasket, if they make it that far (credit to the two keeners who just take out the scalpel blades and get working). Or is the hardest part the first time you must give your classmate an injection? Pushing that 30 millimeter needle through the mucosa, through a stringy pillow of soft tissue, as 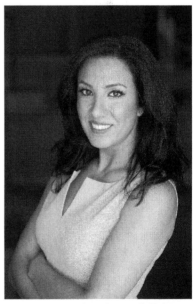 you imagine all kinds of vital structures you're hopefully just passing by. Or is it the first time you have to drill a tooth on a living person? Or the first time you have to surgically extract a tooth, flapping bleeding soft tissue, removing living bone with a 20,000-rpm high speed drill? Or the first time a patient faints in your chair and you're the doctor; you're in charge of figuring out what just happened on the inside of their skin and providing the right emergency care.

The answer is simple. They're all the hardest part. You see, all these challenges have one important thing in common: they are firsts. Every dentist knows each of those feelings because we have all experienced the anxiety of the first time—doing everything we learned—on a human being; kind of like the butterflies of your first kiss; well, not exactly, but you get the idea. We all survive it, but some do better than others. What would make our entire profession better as a whole is if we were taught *how* to survive the toughest times. This has all been done before—and all we must do is learn from history.

The real secret to getting through each step of the way with more ease than you can imagine requires only one thing to always remember to plan with clarity, and that is your personal *growth*. The purpose of this chapter is to teach you another perspective for the regular challenges we face in dentistry, to help you overcome those challenges, and to remind you to recognize and celebrate your accomplishments.

The single most important thing that most young dentists fail to recognize is the need to continue learning. You simply can't see what you don't know, and if you can't see it, you definitely can't treat it. The first step in your journey of personal growth is very much the same; you need to take the time to figure out where you are. Think of a map of the biggest shopping mall you've ever been in and you're trying to find your way to your favorite store. What's the most important thing for you to know so you can get there? You need that red dot that says, "You are here."

You must know where you are in order to be able to get to where you are going. If you are in your first five years of practice, you may be primarily concerned with clinical issues: techniques for better outcomes, larger ranges of treatment options, learning new real-world dentistry skills that you weren't taught in school, and getting better at what you already know. It is crucial after you graduate to realize that the learning has just begun. If you stop learning, you will first be stagnant, and then you will feel you are falling behind. Our profession advances year by year, and there is *much* more to learn than what you learned in school. School formed a baseline, and continuing your education by updating and advancing yourself with CE courses is what will truly make you an excellent clinician. Investing in yourself will give one of the best returns on investment you will ever make in your lifetime.

Now, what happens to a clinician with education and experience? The craft becomes second nature. Comfort comes with clinical experience. You will unconsciously interpret your X-rays, anesthetize your patient, and do your procedures, much like toddlers teetering on their first steps, compared to a child running after a ball in a soccer game, no longer thinking about every step, but now concentrating on the ball and the goal. How long that takes for each person is different, and on average most dentists find five years to be the ticket. At five years of combined continuing education and experience, most dentists no longer feel the anxiety of bread-and-butter dentistry procedures. The best advice I ever received in dentistry was from an amazing teacher who told me to never stop learning. She taught me that if you don't understand something, don't give up—repetition is the key. There are some complex concepts in dentistry and all it takes is repeated exposure for you to become proficient with them. First, you learn everything you can didactically, then you make sure to implement clinically at your pace. You need to see lots of patients and practice as much as you can. Clinical dentistry becomes second nature to you once you are comfortable to the point that your mind doesn't stress and your hands can do it with ease. I promise you, we all get there.

Here's the kicker. Being able to actually practice clinical dentistry requires communication skills. You have to be able to explain to your patients what you see, the whys (why they need it, why it's better to treat than not to treat, risks and benefits, etc.). The best dentists are the ones who communicate so well with patients that the patients come out to reception *asking* for appointments to take care of the recommended treatment. These patients can actually explain exactly what they need and why. You would think this takes a lot of talking on the dentist's part, and while it's true we have to explain diagnoses and treatment to our patients, the best communicators are usually the best listeners. I encourage all dentists to consider communication a key part of the education they are seeking in order to master clinical dentistry. Remember, you will only get the opportunity to do dentistry on willing patients, and those are the ones that have been well-communicated to during treatment planning. The true best path for success is to master your communication and clinical skills, and then tackle the business of dentistry so you are not overwhelmed in every aspect of what you are doing.

When you're ready, there are great benefits to practice ownership. The basis for all the benefits stems from complete control. As an owner, you choose your work hours, your work days, who you want to work with, what types of patients you want to treat, your supplies and materials, your business partners, and so much more on a daily basis. For the seasoned practice owner, generally the initial challenges in clinical dentistry are replaced with clinical confidence, and the biggest challenges for most business owners ensue: finances, staffing, corporate culture, and team alignment.

But wait, when were we ever taught about business?

The truth is, we weren't. Business is foreign to most dentists, and that is what creates the challenges in owing a dental practice. I will tell you that business is a profession of itself, and dentistry is big business. You need to *think like a CEO*. Your business doesn't care that you're a dentist; your business needs to be managed smartly and efficiently. Learn about business. Study other businesses, customer service, target audiences, and marketing.

Think about what you want to do, and find a mentor who is already doing it well. Mentorship is one of the most powerful tools to catapult you to success. Your ideal mentor is someone who excels in their niche and is willing to share generously. Listen to their story, their challenges, their past mistakes, and *learn* from it all. These are invaluable experiences that would take you a lifetime to learn if you tried to go solo. Collaboration is key to success.

Find like-minded people who will tell you the truth. The internet has connected people globally, and you can start there with social media and various online forums that are composed of people in your profession. Find continuing education that resonates with you, and keep on learning. If you find a subject you love, learn everything you can about it from as many sources as you can find. Find a business coach who will be worth their fee exponentially because of what they'll see that you couldn't. Don't go at this alone; you don't have to learn by making *all* of your own mistakes. Of course you will make some, but you don't have to reinvent the wheel. The dental industry is literally thousands of years old, with the first physician of teeth documented in 2600 BC. It is much less painful to learn from the mistakes of others than it is to try to do everything on your own.

One of the pieces of running a business that doesn't come naturally to a lot of people, and causes them a lot of grief before they figure it out, is the leadership piece. You must recognize that your team is one of the most important parts of your practice.

You are the leader of your team. Your energy initiates your practice culture. Your practice vision is what you choose it to be, and your communication of that vision to your team is what makes it a reality. Your team is on a mission to execute your vision. Who those people are is *really* important. The best team members are the ones who are excited about dentistry and care about people. They have an inner motivation for doing their best, they don't want to let the patients or the team down, and they love what they do. If someone hates their job, don't hire them, and don't be afraid to let them go. People create culture, and culture is what your patients feel when they walk into your office.

Once you have the right people in the right roles, you only have to remember one thing every day so you can keep the positive culture you want: people love to feel appreciated. Employees care more about appreciation than they care about money. (I still encourage you to pay them well, as I do believe you get what you pay for.) A very wise businesswoman once told me to appreciate people more than you think they need. Acknowledge their efforts, celebrate their wins, help them through challenges constructively, and for heaven's sake, if you have someone you know is not working out, let them go find their happiness somewhere else. They will thank you for it. A critical part of growing a strong, high-performance, well-managed team is knowing when to hold on to certain people and when to let go of the weakest links.

The reality is we do a *lot*. In our lives, we wear so many hats: we are dentists, we are doctors, we are bosses, we are business owners, we are mothers, we are daughters, we are sisters, we are wives, and so much more. Few professions give people the opportunity to be so much to so many, and still be successful. We can, and we *are* doing this, and we are *good* at it. Many of the best practices in the world are female-run, and we all know our irreplaceable contribution to our families. In the endless pursuit of our endless goals, in our incredible growth mindset, we must remember to occasionally look behind us, measure how far we have come, and celebrate our victories. The personal reward of knowing all you have accomplished creates a sense of fulfillment and gratitude, which are essential components for continued growth and success. "Here's to strong women. May we know them. May we be them. May we raise them." (anonymous).

Dr. Nada Albatish owns and operates a multi-disciplinary comprehensive practice, All Smiles Dental Centre, just north of Toronto. Dr. Albatish is a consummate learner and is committed to advanced continuing education, first by completing a General Practice Residency immediately out of dental school, followed by hundreds of hours of CE each year.

Dr. Albatish's love for complex cosmetic and rehabilitative dentistry has earned her distinction among her peers. She is honored to serve as Faculty for Clinical Mastery Series and as Curator for Restorative Nation online. As a speaker, author, and key opinion leader, Dr. Albatish is inspired by helping her fellow dentists achieve excellence, predictability, and confidence in their craft. She acts as a mentor and support system for clinicians around North America and is committed to the success of others and the advancement of the dental profession at large.

To connect with Dr. Albatish, please contact her at NAlbatish@gmail.com.

Chapter Three
Timing is Everything

As dentists we often have characteristics and personality traits like being in control, perfectionism, and type-A personality, but sometimes we have to remind ourselves that not everything can be in our control. I remember thinking as a teenager that I would be married at 27 or 28 and then have a baby at 29 and another at 31. Little did I know that I wouldn't marry until 32, have my first child at 36 and my second at 38.

I had always wanted my own practice and thought that buying into a partnership was my path. I worked at many different offices as an associate and collected experience in working with other people and learning the business side of dentistry. I definitely knew what I liked and what I did not like about each office I worked in. There were things that I learned working in the dental office as an assistant that I never would have learned in dental school; not just about dentistry itself, but about how people behaved. I've seen the good, the bad, and the ugly. That insight stays with you, and you file it away until you need to use it. Sometimes I have friends who think they need to buy a practice or start a practice when they are in the second trimester but it's just not the right time. It's harder for us women who are moms trying to raise our children and take care of our families and take care of our patients. I was fortunate to start a FFS scratch practice after I got married and before I had kids. My practice was four years old before I had my first child. During those four years, I poured my heart and soul into my practice and made it grow. I worked around the clock and it didn't feel like work because I enjoyed it so much. There was some level of fear from not knowing what I was doing, but there was also the fear of failure and the fear of not making money. I used that fear to fuel myself into success. I grabbed myself by the shoulders and told myself that I had no choice but to sink or swim. And I wasn't going to sink; that was not an option. With that in mind, I had to keep my head above water and I figured things out along the way.

Had I decided to have kids first, I'm not certain I would have started a practice. When you're a first-time mom, there's a learning curve, and there are lots of things you experience that your friends don't tell you. The same is true for a dental practice; there is a learning curve in running a business and things that you experience that other owners may not. I think the Good Lord knew that if I had kids first, I would have shied away from starting a scratch fee-for-service practice. I had the opportunity to start one and I went for it. That was the best decision ever made.

After my husband and I married, we decided to move to California to be closer to my sister, who lived in Laguna Beach. We moved to Newport Coast and I went through the hoops of obtaining a California dental license. Who knew that I would have the most difficult time finding a position as an associate? It was 2008, the economy had turned, and there were not as many opportunities. After five months, we went back to Chicago because three offices that I had worked in wanted me to return. When I got back, I decided I wanted more from my career. I reflected on my life and decided it was time for more. I started out as an assistant and worked my way up the ladder. I approached my boss in Lincoln Park where I'd spent most of my time as an associate and discussed my options of buying into the practice. I told him that after four years of being there, I had built my own book of patients and did my share of marketing his practice and name. I worked hard and wanted to be more than an associate. He told me that I could be 49% and he would be 51%, that he was always going to be the captain of his ship. At that point, I said, "Thank you for the opportunity," and that I'd consider it. There was no way in hell I was going to go for that, so that was it for me; it was my time to leave the nest and be on my own. There were no practices to buy and there was no one that I really wanted to partner with since the other offices I worked at were in the suburbs. The time was now or never; it was *show time*, and I was fired up. For the next eight months, I worked under the radar and kept my lips sealed. My husband and I found the perfect location for my start-up office. He helped me find the right team of experts and away I went. The practice was under construction, and I opened my doors August, 2009. The timing was not right in the perspective of the economy, but somehow by the grace of God, I was shielded from that slump. It was the perfect timing for Yummy Dental & Orthodontics for Kids.

Introducing Dr. Julie Swift

When Grace asked if I would be willing to cover this topic, I gladly accepted, as I am a big believer in the concept of timing, co-incidence, and circumstances aligning if we are paying attention; although, many times when I am in the middle of one of these situations it does not feel like the best outcome is happening. Over the years, I have learned that even when things are not seemingly going the way I want them to, it

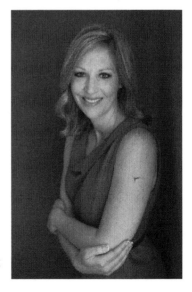

means something even more amazing is just around the corner. The first example of how this played out in my professional life has to do with how I ended up in Topeka, KS. I was the "prepared" second year resident following up with all options as a resident in Dallas, TX. At the same time, I started a long-distance relationship with a young man my UM-KC School of Dentistry friends had set me up with for a formal event that year. Due to our relationship and the fact that he was a teacher and coach in the Kansas City area, I began speaking with colleagues in the KC area. Before the end of second year, I had all but signed on the dotted line to become an associate for a periodontal practice in North Kansas City.

Later that same year, several things happened to upset all of my well-made plans. My then-fiancé decided to take a head coaching position in Topeka, so that meant I would have to commute back and forth from Topeka. That seemed like viable option since we still planned for him to get a job back in Kansas City; the commuting would only be for a year or two. I also started checking with periodontal practices closer to Topeka so that on Friday nights I could attend the football games he would be coaching. I actually arranged my schedule with two practices so that I could alternate working with each one on Fridays. Within six months, all that planning would be for not because the North Kansas City periodontist no longer thought he wanted an associate, and one of the periodontists in Topeka passed away unexpectedly. That meant I would be starting completely over with my search for a job with less than three months to graduation from my residency program. I was disappointed, frustrated, sad, and nervous.

I immediately did two things, as action was needed. I inquired about purchasing the Topeka practice where the periodontist had suddenly passed away. When I could tell that was not going to be possible, I spoke with the owner of the competing practice. I had purposefully not talked with him about working on Fridays as I thought he would want someone for more hours, since he was closer to retirement age. That decision almost cost me as he knew he was my second choice. Even after negotiating terms for me to become his associate, he almost backed out because he was concerned I would not stay in Topeka or be committed to his practice.

All of this took place in 2004. I was his associate for two years and he then became my associate for two years once I took over ownership in 2006. I am in the same practice, although we have moved the office. The only staff member that has stayed with me the entire time is the assistant that was hired specifically for me.

Dr. Stone still comes to deliver Christmas gifts to all of our staff and I could not be more pleased that I ended up in Topeka, as it has been a fantastic place to live, work, and raise my daughter.

Personally, the best example of timing being everything involving how my husband and I met. I'd been divorced from my daughter's dad for about four years. I had gone on sporadic dates and pretty much decided it was not likely I would find a new spouse that wanted an independent, professional woman for a wife and would be a suitable person I wanted to spend the rest of my life with. I'd been disappointed with some of the people that friends had tried to set me up with and online options were not successful in my area.

At the time Brad sent me a friend request on Facebook, I was very leery of accepting "friends" that I did not personally know since I tend to post lots of pictures of my daughter. Typically, I am at least somewhat reassured if we at least have several mutual friends. He and I had one mutual person in common and that was the woman that had taken my most recent professional photo that was used for advertising pieces; therefore, before I accepted his request I did a little more digging into his background. His profile said he was a general and trauma surgeon at one of the local hospitals, so I confirmed that via the hospital web page. I also looked to see if he owned a house within our county and it turned out his house was within blocks of my office location. I decided to go ahead and accept the friend request, knowing that I could unfriend or block him at any time.

He waited a couple of more days then sent me a private message and we began talking thru messenger. In the beginning, he led me to believe that a work colleague had suggested he get to know me and I played along until he referred to me as dainty. That's when I knew he did not know anyone that knew me because I am tall; no one would ever describe my personality as dainty either. That is when he confessed that he had seen my advertisement (with the photo taken by the one mutual friend) in a high-end magazine that is delivered to homes around town. He had thought to himself that there was a professional woman he would like to meet and get to know. He then started checking around to see if I was married or not and what the story was about me. The truly funny part of this story is that I had almost cancelled the ads for that magazine because by then we had established brand recognition and the advertising rates had increased yet again. Thankfully, I decided to keep the advertisements for one more year. Within two years of him seeing my ad, we were engaged and have now been married for almost three years. We now have over 80 mutual friends on Facebook.

Now, these examples both had very positive outcomes, but there have been other incidences in my life where timing led to very negative consequences. The most notable is the car accident that claimed the lives of my sister and her husband back in 1990. It was the Friday night of Labor Day weekend and they were driving to her in-laws' house for dinner. Their truck hydroplaned on the wet roads, and since that stretch of highway was not divided, an oncoming car hit them. If they had left five minutes earlier or later they might not have been on a part of the highway that was undivided or they might not have hit that particular spot to send them spinning in the first place.

That car accident happened at the end of my first college week. For my entire adult life, I have known that everything can change in the blink of an eye. I do not believe in pre-destination and have never believed my sister and her husband would have died at that time no matter what the circumstances were. I do believe that timing of events and/or the way certain circumstances align in our lives do have the potential to dramatically change our lives for the better or worse. Therefore, I believe we must always be looking for the opportunities that are created by sometimes seemingly-bad things falling through and celebrate when even better outcomes happen because we were patient enough to see what might happen instead.

Originally from Wichita, Dr. Swift earned her undergraduate degree from Wichita State University and her Doctor of Dental Surgery degree from the University of Missouri-Kansas City. After a three-year residency, she earned her master's degree and Certificate in Periodontics from Baylor College of Dentistry in Dallas. Dr. Swift, a board-certified Diplomate of the American Academy of Periodontology, has practiced in Topeka since 2004. In 2015, she was inducted as a Fellow in the American College of Dentists. She regularly attends continuing education courses to keep up to date on the latest periodontal and implant procedures.

Dr. Swift is past president of both the Topeka District Dental Society and the Missouri-Kansas Periodontal Association. In 2007, she co-chaired the Kansas Mission of Mercy dental project held at the Kansas Expocentre and helped again when the KMOM was held again in Topeka (2015). Dr. Swift was honored in 2010 as one of Topeka's "20 under 40" and was named to the 2012 Leadership Greater Topeka class. She currently serves on the Topeka Shawnee Country Public Library and the Topeka Community Foundation boards. Dr. Swift spends her time away from work with her husband and daughter and enjoys reading, traveling, and piecing quilts. To connect with Dr. Swift, please contact her at DrSwift@TopekaPerio.com.

Chapter Four
Make Your Own Magic

One important lesson I learned during my time as an associate was that no one was going to just hand me a silver platter with everything I wanted. Practicing as a young associate, even with all that experience as a dental assistant had some challenges. My first position was at a private practice in Lincoln Park, one of Chicago's affluent neighborhoods. The children came in black cars, had cell phones better than mine, came with their nannies. The parents were demanding as hell and did not accept NO for an answer. They made requests that I come in early, before the office opened, so that they could carry on with their day. I even remember moms telling my boss that I wasn't experienced enough or that I wasn't accommodating enough.

These were hard lessons I had to learn that were not explained to me in dental school. Many times, the senior doctor had to take me aside and explain why I had to do things his way and not what I learned in school. I had to learn to work in a team environment and practice accordingly, but as I continued to take the feedback, I began to develop my own style. I learned to communicate effectively with parents and children and meet expectations. My dentistry continued to grow as I learned more orthodontics. As my practice grew within that practice and my patient base grew, I took every chance I could to promote myself. The senior doctor had me going to do school presentations instead of seeing patients during the day. I was angry at him because I felt that it was a waste of my time. Why was I advertising for his practice and not in the office making money? As an associate, you want to make money and you are hungry to see your numbers grow. I mean, isn't that why we wanted to be dentists? After some time and few months, I saw the fruits of my own labor. There was a policy in the office that all new patients had to have their first visit with the owner of the practice. That was fine for a while, but then parents were calling and specifically asking for me. This was my a-ha moment because it was at this time when I finally figured out that I had to make things happen for myself.

I was making my own magic and I learned a hard lesson; even though I wasn't in the office producing, I was learning a lesson in marketing. I was getting my own name out in the community and making a name for myself separate from the practice and separate from my boss. I called all the local schools on my down time and got in for presentations. Back then there was no social media, just email. I had sent out emails to numerous principals of schools, I even told the parents of my patients that I would go to their kids' schools to be the community member and give a presentation about dentistry and nutrition.

Soon, my book of business began to grow and I was getting my name out there. It wasn't long before I was getting many phone calls and appointment requests and filling my own schedule. I felt good about the work I did and was satisfied that I was making my own magic. With a lot of hard work and a little luck, my production numbers grew. It was because I made it happen. I was no longer riding the coat tails of my boss and his brand. The icing on the cake was visiting Lincoln Park Preschool. I played with the kids and gave out goodie bags. I brought a puppet to show three- and four-year-olds how to brush their teeth. Two weeks later, a mom came into the office and asked, "We need to see Dr. Grace! My daughter won't stop talking about her." It is now 2018, and that little girl is still my patient.

It wasn't long before I caught onto what my boss was doing to increase his referrals. He was going to meetings with pediatricians in the area to ask for referrals. He never took me with him; he just spoke about the meetings. I felt intimidated at first, thinking, *Well, none of the owners are going to want to meet me, an associate,* but I put that fear aside and decided that if I was going to get my name out there, I had to make my own magic, scared or not. I took my business cards, bought my own baked goods, and took a day driving around and visiting pediatricians. As I thought, no one had time to meet me in person, but I went anyway and made friends with the front desk. That was the easy part of my day, actually, because it brought me back to when I was in college and sat at the front desk of dental offices. I remembered being in high school, sitting at the reception desk, taking phone calls for my pediatrician. It was my first job in high school, to work in the medical field. I remembered that front desk people have all the power. Everyone filtered through the front desk—patients, sales reps, assistants. The front desk knew everything that went on and had the power to give appointment times to patients they liked and people they liked. I made sure to be very friendly with the front desk so that they knew and remembered me and would refer their patients to me.

I went back every three months with goodies in hand and business cards to give out. It took me some time to figure out that the owners of practices were all about the same age as my boss. There were alliances and relationships formed among the practice owners. Certain pediatricians referred to our competition and certain ones referred to us. It was almost like a monopoly and if you were an associate, you were just tied to the owner. One time, I actually got through the front desk ladies and got to meet with the pediatricians that were on lunch. My very first informal meeting was with Dr. Marc Weissbluth, the very famous sleep doctor. His book, *Healthy Sleep Habits Healthy Babies* is a top seller and he is the expert on that topic. I walked into the communal doctor's office and there he was, looking very dapper and doctor-like with his spectacles. I brought my box of cookies and introduced myself to him and handed him my cookies. He looked me up and down with favor, thank goodness I was well dressed and groomed that day, and he smiled and shook my hand. He then looked at the box of Dinkel's cookies and said, "Very good taste in bakeries." I couldn't believe that he even knew what Dinkel's was; it is a famous bakery in Chicago. He then introduced me to his associates who were my cohorts. I took the opportunity to get to know them and exchange emails. I began to form friendships with two of the associates who worked for Dr. Weissbluth. Fast-forward to 2011, they along with the other associates bought the practice and Marc retired; my point being, I had cultivated the relationships with those that were eventually going to take over. I was building my own relationships and building my own network.

An Interview with Dr. Gina Dorfman

1. How long have you been a dentist? How long have you owned your own business?

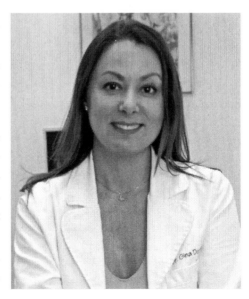

I graduated from USC School of Dentistry in 2000 and have been in private practice for 17 years now. Initially, I worked as an associate and started my dental practice from scratch in Canyon Country, CA in 2002. We just celebrated our 15-year anniversary.

2. What is the reason you wanted to be a dentist?

My grandmother was a medical doctor in Russia. I've always admired her strength and courage. I marveled how she managed to do so much and make everything appear effortless. I was proud of how respected and loved she was by her patients, co-workers, and friends. I considered a career in medicine, but I was also interested in owning my own business one day. The idea of building something that can work and be profitable when I am not around really appealed to me. I've always wanted to have a family and children, and I wanted to make sure that my career allows me the opportunity to be present both at work and at home. Ultimately, I chose dentistry because dentistry seemed to have a more streamlined pathway to practice ownership.

3. How did you make your own magic?

I didn't know I was making my own magic, at least I wasn't intentional about it at first. I knew exactly what I wanted to accomplish in life and I had a plan. I had a strong work ethic, and I wasn't afraid of working hard and takings risks. I just kept plugging along, doing more, learning, and making improvements. By 2009, I was happily married, owned two busy dental practices, and had two adorable and healthy children. I worked four days clinically, managed 30 employees, and just set out to start a dental software company with my dad and my husband. On a surface, I was successful; I was making a great living, having fun, and accomplishing a lot, but I also felt thinly stretched and stressed. I knew I could just stay up another hour and have another cup of coffee in the morning to get more done, but I started to realize that burning midnight oil is not a good long-term strategy. I knew that I was neglecting my health and my sanity and that trying to be a super-woman was not a sustainable strategy. I started to worry that my life will just flash in front of my eyes. I heard a quote by Allen Saunders who said: "Life is what happens while you are busy making other plans," and I thought that this quote applied to me perfectly. It was time for a change. It was time to design the life I wanted to live, so I set out on a journey of self-discovery and research. I've read a lot of great time-management books, including books by Steven Covey, Brian Tracy, and David Allen. I've learned that making time to concentrate on things that are important but not urgent is critical. I've learned that I should focus my energy and time on the things that I do best and delegate everything else. I've taken a Kolbe test, and I've learned about my strengths. Fortunately, my strengths turned out to be well-suited for creating a vision and an implementation strategy. I've also learned to identify other people's strengths and how to coordinate these strengths for our mutual growth.

To be quite honest, I am still a busy mom. This will never change, but my life is more deliberate and more satisfying. More importantly, I have more time for my family and myself. I am also more forgiving of myself. I know I am getting the important stuff done and I don't worry when the little things don't get done or don't come out perfect.

4. What other business ventures have you started? Why did you decide to partner up in YAPI?

Starting a software company was never a part of the plan, but now that I understand myself better, I understand how it happened. My why—my motivation to get out of bed in the morning—is to improve things. I cannot help myself. I am always asking, *How can we do this better?*

When I started my practice, I became obsessed with efficiency. I believed that if I had sound office systems, I could hire smart people with great attitudes and train them easily. I set out to create simple, reproducible systems. I've designed, implemented, tweaked, and revised my business processes and procedures until I felt I was able to eliminate any unnecessary steps and simplify everything else. I wanted to build a paperless ecosystem, improve team communication, automate repetitive tasks, and organize office workflows. In the process, I've come up with a long list of things that I wished my practice management software could do. Eventually, I turned to my dad, a veteran software engineer, for help. My dad had just recently retired and was already showing the signs of boredom.

As I shared my ideas, he asked a lot of his usual "What's the point?" questions. The next morning, he showed me something that would turn out to be our next business venture. YAPI began as a simple intra-office communication software. As we implemented YAPI in my practice, my team and I started to come up with more ideas and my dad never looked bored again. I showed YAPI to a few friends, and they loved it. One of them posted about YAPI on DentalTown. The response was overwhelming. In 2011, we introduced YAPI at the Townie meeting in Las Vegas and signed our first 11 customers. By the end of our first year, we had 75 customers. Building a software company was a great adventure that allowed me to travel, meet a lot of great people, and work with my family. Now, six years later, we have over 30 employees and thousands of customers.

5. What is the best piece of advice you can give to another mommy dentist in business?

First and foremost, let go of the guilt. Many of us tend to live with a perpetual guilt that we are neglecting our responsibilities. We feel guilty when we take time off work to be with our families, and we feel guilty that we are not there for the family when we put extra time into our work and our businesses. We are in search of life-work balance, but we forget that life-work balance does not exist. Nothing in the universe is ever in balance; some days our family needs us more and other days our work requires more of our focus. Instead of seeking balance, strive for presence. Choose the quality over quantity and be fully present in every activity. Don't fold laundry next to your kids—get down on the floor and play with them.

Learn your strengths and spend your time on activities where your strengths shine.

Allocate time for the rocks—the big important tasks that will bring the most value to your life. Block the time on your schedule when you will work on the projects that will make a difference. Sprinkle the busy work around your big rocks (Stephen Covey).

Don't feel bad asking for help. In fact, rely on other people's strengths to help you get more done. Learn to delegate. Ask yourself: "Am I the best person to be doing this?" If not, find the right person and delegate. Delegation is quite simple: envision the final result, find the right person with the skills required to accomplish it, communicate what the final result will look and feel like, explain the purpose and the goal, and get out of the way. Concentrate on things that are important to you or that you are good at and delegate everything else. Hire someone to fold your laundry. I haven't held an iron in years, and I haven't missed it. I owe every single ounce of my success to my family and friends who supported and helped me, my peers who generously shared their ideas, and my loyal and hardworking employees who make the magic possible.

Surround yourself with successful and positive people. Surround yourself with people who want you to succeed and will pull you up, not weigh you down.

Learn to say NO. Growing up, we learned to be nice and play well with others. We learned to be helpful, and therefore, we often say YES to things that we don't want to do or don't have time for because we don't want to disappoint people.

Make your magic. Envision the life you want to live and reverse engineer your vision to come up with actionable steps you need to take to accomplish them. Place some milestones, celebrate every accomplishment.

Take great care of yourself. My mother-in-law always says, "Above all, your kids need healthy parents."

Stand up for yourself; speak up and ask for what you need from others. We often don't advocate for ourselves because we don't want to come off as self-aggrandizing or be called a bitch, but when we don't expect our spouses to step up and share our family responsibilities or when we don't expect our employees to respect us as they would our male counterparts, we get the short end of the stick. You get what you expect. Expect more.

For almost two decades, Dr. Gina Dorfman has continually proved herself to be an innovative leader in the field of dentistry. As a dentist, practice owner, and entrepreneur Dr.

Dorfman has had the opportunity to engage with dental professionals across the country with the goal of helping them grow and thrive. Graduating from the University of Southern California in 1996 and earning a degree in Biochemistry, Dr. Dorfman completed her dental training at the Herman Ostrow School of Dentistry in 2000, and shortly after started her practice near Los Angeles.

While starting a practice in a saturated market came with challenges, the practice has grown tremendously, expanding to several locations. With her experience running multiple practices and leading a big team, Dr. Dorfman has developed a unique insight into how efficient practices organize and operate and how dental teams can work together to overcome obstacles and reach their goals. Dr. Dorfman has presented at multiple local and national dental meeting, such as the Townie Meeting and Practice on Fire Live. Recently, she had the honor of joining the faculty at the Dental Success Network, a unique community dedicated to advanced learning and collaboration.

Dr. Dorfman is also a frequent contributor to several industry blogs and the host of Behind the Smiles vlog that features the most disruptive and influential members of the dental community who are moving dentistry forward. Dr. Dorfman spends many hours in continuing education each year to further her expertise and is on the cutting edge of technology.

Her passion for creating systems and leveraging technology to streamline practice operations is what led her to co-found YAPI, a robust dental practice automation software, where she currently serves as COO of the company.

When she is not working, Dr. Dorfman enjoys hiking, reading and spending time with her husband Ken, their two children, Mila and Lenny, and a dog named Axel. To connect with Dr. Dorfman, contact her at DrGina@YAPICentral.com or www.YAPIapp.com.

Chapter Five
Coulda, Woulda, Shoulda

It's easy to live in that mindset—to think, *I should have done that*, but instead, I did something else. Or instead of saying one thing to the patient, I should have said something else. We all have had moments where we drive home for 30 minutes conjuring up all the things we could have said and done, but the past is the past. There are not enough hours in the day to dwell on the past. We must focus on the future and learn from the past. It's not like me to regret many choices; I am a decisive person and pretty set on my goals, but when I find myself thinking about the past, I remember the lesson I learned and move forward. The only area in my life that I could think of that I do regret is not starting my family sooner. I was married in 2008 at the age of 32. It was definitely not what I had planned and definitely not the appropriate age by Korean standards. I was considered an old maid whose ship had sailed. My own father told me to move back home with him and my mother. No thank you! I had lived a life of a student, going to school full time, and not having much opportunity to find the right person. Either that or I was dating the wrong person and found myself stuck in the wrong relationship. It was 2003 and I was in my pediatric residency dating a guy that was perfect in my mind. We dated a long time and before I knew it we had broken up and gotten back together several times. In 2006, we broke up for good and I was heartbroken, not just because of a failed relationship, but because I thought that he was the one. I remember waking up in my studio apartment staring at the ceiling with a tear running down my cheek. It was my 30th birthday and I was alone as a single woman. According to my plan, I was two years late in getting married, and I was panicked. I went through so many mixed emotions and I finally got to the point later in the year that I accepted my age and single life. I decided it was better to be happy and alone than to be miserable and with someone who was going to string me along. It wasn't until then that I had met my now-husband, who is perfectly suited for me. It's funny how God works in mysterious ways and teaches us lessons along the way. Had I not gone through the bad times, I wouldn't be able to appreciate the good times.

Now, going back to being married for four years, my husband, Kent and I had the best time being married. We truly enjoyed ourselves and although we didn't have much money at that time, we knew how to have a good time. The marital bliss of being newlyweds swept us off of our feet and onto so many adventures. We travelled all over far and wide and enjoyed just getting to know each other. One of my favorite hobbies is to travel and so we did just that. We went to Asia, Canada, Europe, Australia, and all over the U.S. During that time, we opened the first Yummy Dental for Kids. One year after we were married, my dream of being a practice owner came into fruition. I poured my blood, sweat, and tears into my business. As a pediatric dentist working with children all day every day, my body never went into a biological-clock mode. I was fulfilled seeing my pediatric patients every day and coming home to my husband and our perfectly clean and quiet apartment. About three years later, we started to discuss the possibility of starting a family. We looked at each other and hemmed and hawed about not being able to travel anymore and needing a bigger space. Kent and I were nervous that our lifestyles of being DINK's would be over (dual income no kids). We went through the advantages and disadvantages of having children, or at least one child, and decided that maybe we should have one because otherwise who was going to take care of us in our old age?

I remember clear as day, the autumn night we were out to dinner at Dee's, our local favorite Chinese restaurant. We sat in the back booth where the tablecloth had white paper over it. I asked our server, Jade, for a pen and then mapped out when I wanted our first child to be born. I explained to Kent that I needed to have the baby born, if at all possible during the winter months when the practice was slow. We wrote out all the months of the year and I circled December, January, and February, then we counted backwards nine to 10 months and circled February, March, and April. Now, I was on a mission, just like I had planned out all the details of my business, I was going to plan out all the details of pregnancy, down to the gender.

Like marriage, I was one of the last ones to get married amongst my friends and of course, the last to have children. I gathered as much information as I could from them and from all the mothers that brought their kids to my practice. This information was truly gold. I had doubts of getting pregnant right away because I worked with nitrous oxide and also because many of my dentist friends went through in vitro or alternate kinds of medicine to conceive. The best piece of advice my friends gave me was to start acupuncture and to prepare my body for conception, so I made my appointment in November and consulted with the acupuncturist. She altered my diet and gave me herbal supplements to take to help my "chi" blood flow. I loved going once a week and sleeping on a warm table, albeit needles sticking out of me. It was relaxing and a great way to make my body prepare for the most life-changing experience. Kelly Lee, the owner of the business, told me to prepare for three months and that I would notice changes in my body, but it would take three months. I did just that and I started to follow other instructions from other people like tracking ovulation on my iPhone app and listening to moms about which ovulation kits were the best and most accurate. One of the best pieces of advice was to keep testing ovulation after day 11 because some women ovulated way late like day 18 or 19. Literally, in March and after three months of acupuncture and ovulation kits, I decided it was time to try, and of course, I had to research how to get pregnant with a girl. I just needed to have a daughter in my life. I grew up with one sister and never had a brother, so for me to have a son would feel so awkward. After researching what foods to eat and when to make a "deposit," we became pregnant on our first try. That month, I was so tired and I kept drinking coffee to stay awake. My expectation was that it would take at least six months, but when I missed my period, I was stunned. Could I have really gotten pregnant on our first attempt? Kent and I went to the drugstore and bought two kits, went straight home, and yes, it was certain that we were pregnant. I fell to my knees, praying thankfully for this beautiful blessing; we were shocked and overjoyed.

Now, no one really ever prepares you about pregnancy and how difficult it can be, but I had a rough pregnancy. I had morning sickness and every symptom in the book. I continued with acupuncture and it helped immensely with that sickness, but I never understood why it was called morning sickness when I felt sick *all the time*. There were days that I had to just lie down under my desk at my office and sleep. After three months of not telling anyone, we were so excited to share the news. My patients were ecstatic that I was now becoming one of them and crossing over. Many of my patients thought that I already had kids and that I had a family of 10.

Fast forward four years. I not only have a four-and-a-half-year-old daughter, I also have a three-year-old son. He was planned out just like my first born. I wanted him to arrive at the end of August, after everyone was in school, of course. I wanted him to be a summer baby, opposite his sister winter baby, just like me and my sister.

Now, if I only knew how difficult it is to raise children and how physically exhausting it is and how hard it is to bounce back, I would have started to have children at a younger age. I think that is my personal coulda, woulda, shoulda, and being over 40 years old, my advanced maternal age is not something I want to mess with. At this point, I feel there are too many potential downsides to having another child, but had I started at a younger age, I think I woulda had a third child; however, had I started a family at a younger age, my practice may not be where it is now, and I am grateful that I had that time to pour my heart and soul into my business before pouring my heart and soul into my kids.

An Interview with Dr. Wendy Xue

1. Is there anything in your life you wish you had done differently?

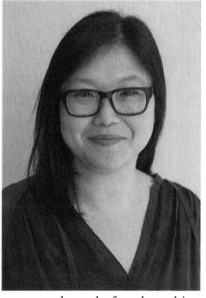

Gosh, I think if anyone says no, they are lying. There's a reason that the famous saying, "Hindsight is 20-20" exists. Of course, there are things I wish I could have done differently. One of the biggest things would be opening my practice earlier. I never felt quite ready, and always felt I had more to learn before launching my own brand; however, I now realize that there is no such thing as feeling 100% ready. Starting a practice takes quite a leap of faith as there is no way to control everything. Realizing this sooner would have brought me to the current stage of practice sooner. The other thing I wish I could change would be starting a family earlier. The female body is such an amazing thing, and we have been blessed to create and grow babies, but this body is so different in our twenties versus thirties versus forties. Under ideal timing, I would have had children in my twenties, started the practice in my thirties, and enjoyed the fruits of my labor forties and on. That being said, I think the stairs make the ladder. I have no regrets, and without all of the steps (and missteps), I would not be the person, mother, or doctor I am today.

2. How do you feel about regrets? What is the best way to avoid being regretful?

I don't do regrets. That may sound trite, but that is how I live my life. To regret means to dwell—on mistakes and failures. Learn from your mistakes and move on. Life is too short for regret. There are lessons to be learned from things that make us regret, but there is so much more value in being able to grow from those difficult situations and evolve into the next stage of you. I read a great article not too long ago that highlights the reasons why some children are more likely to succeed. One of those differences is how children deal with failure. Carol Dweck, a Stanford University psychologist, has discovered that "children (and adults) think about success in one of two ways. One is called a fixed mindset, which assumes that our character, intelligence, and creative ability are static and cannot change in any meaningful way, and success is the affirmation of that inherent intelligence. On the other hand, a growth mindset thrives on challenge and sees failure not as evidence of unintelligence but as a heartening springboard for growth and for stretching our existing abilities." It has been said that if kids are told they have done well because of their innate intelligence and ability, a fixed mindset is created; however, if children are taught that they succeeded due to effort, a growth mindset is taught.

I think as strong, multi-tasking women, we must develop a growth mindset. We need to be able to forgive ourselves as well. We all know mommy guilt a bit too well, but to truly understand that each and every mistake will only lead to a better, more successful future will keep the regret away. I guess to truly avoid regret, we all need to come from a place of kindness; to ourselves, our family—especially our children—our staff, and even strangers. Living a life of love will be the ultimate prevention of regret because often we regret due to the harshness of our actions.

3. Do you ever have moments where you say: "I should have, I could have, I would have"?

Gosh, doesn't everybody? I guess this question goes hand in hand with the ones regarding regret. I try not to dwell on what should have, could have, or would have been, instead looking at the current path and focusing more on what *will* be.

I think being a Christian and having faith in a Savior has a lot to do with being able to look at the future instead of the past. God makes me see that everything happens according to His will, and I am blessed to have a hand in making that *will* come alive.

Being a mother also doesn't allow much room for wondering what could have been. I think having a child forces us to look past the possibilities and seek the realities; the realities which will help our families grow and flourish.

4. What is the best piece of advice for those you mentor?

Every day that one can be a doctor, a mother, a wife, and a daughter is a gift. Treat every challenge or obstacle as an opportunity to learn, grow, and mature. If you are currently an associate, be hungry. No one teaches us about the struggles of business in school, so keep your eyes open and practice with intentions to build, even if you do not own the practice, because *you* are your brand and your brand will follow you wherever you go. Be kind and helpful to your mentors because some knowledge cannot be learned from books.

Be humble and practice with empathy. We have all been given a gift where we can use our knowledge and clinical skills to help and cure others. This gift is to be treated with respect and to be given to others even when they cannot necessarily afford it. Kindness is the best testament to your reputation, and that is what will make you a successful business woman.

Dr. Wendy Xue was born in Shanghai and came to America at the age of nine. Dr. Xue grew up on the East Coast, but developed a love for other cultures through traveling abroad with her family almost every summer. She attended Cornell University, and worked in non-profit for during her gap year before moving on to Columbia University where she obtained her Degree of Dental Surgery. Dr. Xue has always had a passion for working with children so naturally progressed into the specialty of pediatric dentistry. Dr. Xue has been practicing pediatric dentistry or more than years and owns a practice in NYC.

The best part of being business owner is the flexibility, which is a very important thing for the modern working mother. Dr. Xue understands the challenges associated with wearing the hats of motherhood, doctor and wife, and is one of the main reasons she wanted to contribute to this book. In her spare time, she loves to travel with her family and spends as much time as she can with her girlfriends. To connect with Dr. Xue, please contact her at DrWendy@wxdds.com.

Chapter Six
Dating Your Spouse, Your Friends, and Yourself

How often do you make time for yourself, your spouse, or your friends? I am a very social creature and love to meet new people and see my friends, but once I began my business, time was not of the essence. I was so wrapped up in my work that I just stopped seeing friends. All I had time was for my business and my own personal time, like exercising and going out with my husband. I had time for personal matters like getting my hair done and nails, going to doctor's appointments, and esthetic types of treatments like massages and facials, but once my first child came along it seemed like all of that went out the window. My husband and I promised each other that we would have babysitters every weekend so we could go out for dinner and we have kept that promise to each other. It was a great way to date each other and still feel like we weren't always with our kids. I still made time for working out, but slowly all the other things began to be a distant memory. I was running around with my hair up in a ponytail and barely had makeup on. I remembered to brush my teeth but some days it seemed like that was it. After the second child, it was harder to even add exercise to the schedule, but one thing was for certain; I could count on my trusty yoga teacher to come once or twice a week for a private session.

Being a dentist is a very physically demanding job that no one really understands unless they're in the field. I knew early on the importance of exercising and stretching so as to not get injured on the job. All dentists know that back, neck, arm, shoulder, and hips are all parts of the body that can be strained, and quite frankly, can get very injured if under too much stress. I was introduced to chiropractic early in my career and dated a chiropractor and saw immediate benefits of being a patient. I was very religious about stretching in order to preserve my years as a practicing dentist. Even now, I go for maintenance and adjustments to keep from injury. If you don't take the time to care for yourself, your body can and will give out on you.

I know that in my household I am the primary caregiver. That means that I am really responsible for running the household and my children. Often, I think that managing *their* calendars and activities is so much harder than mine. I have two nannies and a personal assistant to help me run the house and get my kids to where they need to be. My husband has a demanding schedule and often he is jet setting around the world consulting large law firms or he is in a tv studio filming for a segment as a legal analyst. Because we have grueling work schedules and a team of people to help us, we often go out to dinner during the weekdays, if he is home, and every weekend. We make it a point to have evening sitters lined up so that we can relax and date each other and date our friends. It's important to have nights to yourself so that your whole life isn't about business and kids. Even when my husband is gone, I will put my kids down for bed and then head out later to have dinner by myself or go get a massage. Living in Chicago, we have so many late-night options that it is easy to find appointments and friends to go out with. There is a never-ending list of restaurants to try and plays to watch or places to get manicures, although there are plenty of nights I stay home and relax with a nice glass of red wine. And there are a few nights that I will venture out and have dinner by myself with no child or adult to interrupt my thoughts. About two times a year, my husband and I will try to get away, just us, without the kids for one or two nights. Luckily, my parents live close by and can stay and watch the kids. It's a wonderful way for us to go and enjoy ourselves and remind us how we used to be before kids. I know that some moms have a hard time leaving their kids at home, but I think it's so important to have that time away as a couple. We pick destinations that are relatively close-by and since Chicago is in the Midwest, we have many options. Kent and I love going to New York because there is just so much to do and see, and of course, *eat*. We recently went to Toronto and had a lovely visit and checked out some major restaurants. Whatever it is that keeps you connected and whatever you did as a couple before kids, it's equally important to enjoy those things after kids.

As mommy dentists in business, we know that it can be very lonely at the top. I often think that no one can understand the demands of our lives besides a mom and a dentist business owner. It is still not the same as being a mom and a dentist that works for someone else. There is a whole different level of responsibility and stress that comes with being an owner of a small business. It's necessary to find support from spouses, friends, and colleagues so that we don't feel isolated. There is comfort in being united with others that are in the same boat, but it's equally important to maintain friendships with our girlfriends that aren't dentists or business owners or even married. My girlfriends all agree that our husbands seem to have more guys' nights out than we do and that they even have more guy trips. As a working mom, I want to see my kids when I can and I want to see them before bed, and even if I do want to go out, I'm just too tired from the day or end of the week.

An Interview with Dr. Shakila Angadi

1. Many moms or wives lose themselves. Why is it so important to take time for yourself?

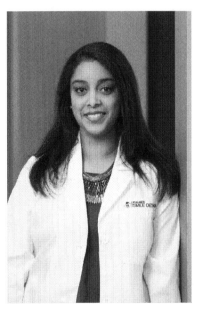

As moms, we take on a lot. We acquire so many sets of expectations, which come in the form of ti-tles—mom, boss, dentist, business owner. I think we have so much to give that we end up losing ourselves in the day-to-day motions of fulfilling all of the obli-gations externally. This leads to burnout, chronic stress, and depletion in ourselves. This is why self-care is the very thing we need to make a conscious effort to keep practicing, as it replenishes who we are as people, and not the titles that we acquire.

2. Why do women and/or moms feel guilty when they do something nice for themselves?

I think we as moms place our happiness and priority on the needs and/or wants of others and equate that to suc-cess in those relationships. The problem with this is that when we don't place ourselves first we cannot fulfil our own needs or desires and feel anxious and depleted.

3. Is it important to go on date nights with spouses?

Super important. More importantly, always making time to do things that are spontaneous, fun, and interactive to build the connection in our relationships. Just because we go out to dinner doesn't automatically lead to connection. It's the novelty, curiosity, and playfulness that we build our relationships on, which is what we want to return to when we spend time with each other.

4. How do relationships dissolve and what can one do to strengthen what they have?

I think relationships dissolve due to a lack of connection. We often miss speaking in the emotional capacity of the other person, which is what emotionally connects us. For instance, many guys find themselves connecting when we do something for them, many women find it more connecting to be reaffirmed. I am a big believer of speaking in each other's love languages and it helps us connect. The other thing we need to do is reflect the emotions in the conversations we have. What is our spouse truly trying to say, what are the emotions behind the words? If we can identify this, we can choose our response better and connect deeper.

5. It seems to me that men don't have a hard time with guys' nights out or even guys' trips, but women have less nights out and less trips. Why is that?

Women tend to place happiness in their titles, as I mentioned above. We often think the world will collapse if we are not in it, when frankly, the moment we take the time for ourselves to go on trips or outings, we can recalibrate with who we are to become happier people. Happier women make happier moms.

6. What do you recommend for us MDIBs to do to refill our tanks and re-energize ourselves?

Self-care and working on a happiness list. Making a list of things that make us happiest, whether it is a good book, cooking, activities, massages, singing, drawing, connecting with friends, etc., we need to know who we are to re-energize ourselves maximally. I personally love anything creative, as it strengthens that part of our mind to come up with solutions down the line.

7. What advice do you have for any mommy dentist in business regarding spending more time on relationships?

Think about the quality of time we place. Do we just exist? How do we feel in them? What do we want to feel more of and how do we change what we are doing right now to do more of that? I think when we take the time to reflect upon how we want to feel, we can create the plans to get to that emotion and holding our relationships accountable for that change. It's constant work, but so fulfilling when we can be satisfied on an emotional level. Spending time doing things we haven't done in our relationships create emotional memories, which cement in the mind more permanently than just spending time.

Dr. Shakila Angadi is a dentist and social and emotional intelligence certified coach located in Charlotte, NC that is determined to help improve the lives of fellow dental professionals. With multiple projects on various platforms, from The Inspired Life Dental podcast to writing for various publications to educating dental professionals, her message to emphasize self-care and promote empathetic communication is clear. With her focus on coaching, she has helped dentists embrace their own EQ to better manage the leadership mindset and increase happiness both in and out of the operatory.

As a mother, dentist, and wife her journey stems from the deep understanding of emotional well-being as a necessity to achieve balance in her personal and professional life. After practicing dentistry for over 11 years, with almost six years in ownership, Dr. Angadi realized that empathetic communication and self-awareness techniques were the key to expanding her practice exponentially, and reducing stress and burnout as a business owner and clinician. After being coached by the leaders in dentistry and emotional intelligence, she was determined to expand her professional expertise to combine the two. As a certified S+EI coach, she bridges the gap between professionalism and emotional agility, and tailors her programs specifically for dentists. Learn more about the EQ programs for dentists on Facebook and Instagram @TheInspiredDentist or contact Dr Angadi at Shakila@The-InspiredDentist.com.

Chapter Seven

Nannies, Babysitters, Daycares ... Oh My!

Okay, this topic is always a hard one for moms. As business owners, we do have options to bring our infants to our work place and set up a room as a nursery. I have always wanted to do that, but I just never had the space in my office for a nursery. In addition, as a pediatric dentist, my office is filled with kids who carry who-knows-what in their little bodies. Someone once said that they are walking pea tree dishes filled with bacteria. And yes, I have over the years caught all the bugs you can think of, even hand foot mouth, which is a childhood disease, so bringing my babies to my office with a nanny was never an option. My mother and father helped out with my first born and were my official nannies for 14 months. My husband and I were forever grateful for that because we could work without any worries about our daughter. This allowed me to return to work without feeling nervous, which was a big deal. I mean, who could be better than your own mother to watch your child? This all worked out wonderfully until one day my poor mother became too tired chasing after a walking toddler who was curious about the whole world. My daughter was as busy as a bee, getting into every cabinet and drawer you could imagine. At that time, I hired a part time student to help my mom watch my 14-month-old daughter. That was the first time I had a non-family member watch my child. I didn't really know where to look, so I posted on my church website and put out feelers on Facebook to see if anyone had any leads. Kelly was our first sitter and she was a student at Moody Bible Institute. She was about 23 and newly married. Her husband and she were wanting to start a family and soon enough she became pregnant. The timing was terrible because then my sister became pregnant and my mother began preparing me for her absence, as she intended to leave to help her in California with her first child. That gave me and my husband anxiety as we would need to truly find a professional nanny, so the search was on again and we asked all of our friends and we cast a wide net in order to find our nanny. We just couldn't find one and the timing was not right. We decided that we would post on Care.com and Sittercity.com, which are two very popular websites for finding caregivers. We were glad to see that they would do the legwork and do the background checks if you paid for them and we were also glad to see that other people put up reviews of them. It was funny to us that we had to create a profile page of our family and post our family photos and list what we were looking for. We thought it was very similar to match.com, which is how we met. Since time was of the essence, we finally decided after multiple interviews that we would hire a Chinese nanny. She was so lovely and we just adored her. She cooked, cleaned, had great availability, had an adult child, and was willing to travel with us. Her English wasn't all that great, but somehow, we managed to communicate. During that time, we had sold our home so quickly that we couldn't find a house to our liking, so we moved to a rental unit. It was at that time that I became pregnant with my second child and also expanded Yummy Dental. What made me decide to do a second office was because my patients were starting to move out of the city and to the suburbs. Many families were complaining about not having enough space and paying for private school for their children. In one summer, 30 of my families moved to the north suburbs where I grew up, so I contacted one of my attendings from my pediatric program whose wife practiced in Glenview. I asked if I could rent her office space once or twice a month to see my patients and to see if they would indeed follow me. For one year, I commuted up north and did a trial run, and it was worth doing, but I knew about six months in that I really wanted to build another location, especially in my hometown, where I grew up. Kent and I had planned on moving to the suburbs, and so I thought that it would be ideal to have this location, especially since the kids would grow up fast and I wanted my office to be near them. I would then cut back on the city location and have associates work for me.

After being comfortable with our new nanny and my mother leaving for California, that comfort of knowing that my kid was ok at home wasn't 100% assured. I trusted my nanny, but I still felt the need to check in two or three times a day. I didn't want to install cameras either because I thought that would make things worse for me. Knowing myself, I'd want to check the cameras constantly, but work was hectic enough that I almost didn't have the time to worry incessantly. I knew that my daughter was in good hands, just not my mother's hands. The year 2013 was epic for me because not only was I pregnant with my second child, I was building out my second scratch office, and building my product business. My husband and I were working on a project called "Dr. Yum's Baby Teeth Cleaners" which took up so much time. He hired another person to help with that business, but we just didn't have the time to really invest in it. I wanted to have something on the market for infant oral health care and developed a swab that had xylitol solution in it to clean the gums and teeth for six months to 2 years of age. It was meant for nursing mothers to help prevent nursing and bottle decay. We were getting traction and sold on Amazon which was a great platform. We tried to get into big box stores and drug stores but it was very difficult and they did not pay very well. We did get into local stores that were happy to promote us, but again that was hard to get into. Finally, we figured out that Amazon was the best platform for us to sell our product. As we were building momentum, so was my husband's business, and the time he put into the product line was starting to compete with his work so much that he really could not focus on it, as his work was far more lucrative. My pregnancy and city office along with the build out caused me to have to put a pause on the product line. While all this was going on, my nanny started to have health issues and needed time off to go to the hospital. She was losing weight rapidly and started to look weak and frail.

My son was induced on August 22nd, so I felt that I had some time to find a replacement while on maternity leave. We couldn't afford to not have a nanny at home and really didn't want our child in day care, so we started the search again. This time, we decided that we were not going to use the online services, as we realized that nannies online didn't have anyone to be accountable to. We thought that a nanny from a friend or someone we knew would be much better than someone online, so we pursued all of our friends one more time and finally found a winner. One of my friends that I grew up with recommended her to me because her children were now in school full time and her nanny raised her two kids; in fact, I had met her before at my office because she brought them in for dental visits. She was working as a nanny for four kids at someone else's house and couldn't handle it. The timing was perfect and she started with me right away. She came to train with Annie and she fit in perfectly. Not only was she healthy, capable, intelligent, and really sweet, she was a perfectionist like me. I was in heaven. She didn't just clean the bottles, she *cleaned* the bottles. She was always punctual and she was always deferential to me and Kent and what we wanted. My friend, Josephine, raved about her and told me that she couldn't trust anyone but her and her husband. I knew that Josephine travelled a lot for work and also had grueling hours, so her word was gold to me. I knew that my new nanny would be awesome, and in fact so awesome, I often tell my husband that she is my "wife." Having a nanny that you can trust to help raise your kids is so crucial to my work life. She helps me stay organized at home so that when I do come home I can spend time with my kids.

I only took a four-week maternity leave with my daughter, so I took six weeks with my son. I had my night nurse ready to go and she stayed with me for four months, which again was money well spent so that I could rest during the night and go to work nice and alert. Once I was back to work, it was business as usual, and we were getting ready to open the second location. We were hitting all the right markers and were going to open on time in December. I wanted to take advantage of the winter vacation that the kids had and also the end of the year insurance benefits running out. I was working longer than usual hours to make this happen and when we had our grand opening, it was so special. All of our Glenview patients that came to see us at the rental office came in to see our new fantastic space.

As the winter passed and summer came, we were ready to make a move to a bigger space. My husband and I decided that we weren't ready to move to the suburbs yet and that we should find a house in the city. Luckily, we found the perfect house for us and moved in October to the best neighborhood we could find. The location was perfect for my commute to both offices and since Kent worked from home when not on the road, he was happy with his own private office. We both realized that with him on the road so much, I needed to be close to where the kids are; not only that, I needed more help. The new house was overwhelming for me. Where was I going to find the time to book contractors and clean and do all the things needed for home ownership? It was then that we decided we needed a house manager that could also serve as a caregiver to our children. This new territory was nothing that we had experienced before, so we went straight to the professionals and paid a large fee, but it was money well spent. I researched several agencies that placed nannies and house managers, but I finally went back to a nanny agency that I had met at an event that we were co-hosting for marketing purposes. She was an amazing help and knew exactly what I was looking for. She asked my specific needs and then helped me find Taylor, a Columbia University graduate with a degree in early childhood education. She was a kindergarten teacher from New York and had moved to Chicago to be closer to family. Taylor was a dream come true because I knew that she could handle our needs, but also because our oldest daughter was going to need some teacherly love at home.

Between her and Martha, our nanny, we had all our needs covered; they did the grocery shopping, dry cleaning, house repairs and maintenance, post office runs, picked up kids from preschool, went to activities—you name it they did it. Without them, I would not be able to do what I do best and that is to run my two dental offices and see my patients. Now, don't get me wrong, on my days off, I do take my kids to activities and play dates. I am able to best spend quality time with them if I don't have to worry about all the other day-to-day things. Again, I have learned to delegate so that I can be with my family and have that quality time with them, like being a chaperone on their field trips.

People ask me all the time, "Wouldn't you rather have an au pair at your house so that you don't have to find babysitters at night?" My response is always no. I have heard one too many stories about live-in nannies from other countries and the nightmare it is to get them out. Other colleagues of mine that have had au pairs have had multiple who have stolen from them, haven't done what they were supposed to, and were just plain young. For me, I just don't have the personality to have a stranger live in my house; it's just too awkward for me. I don't like the feeling that there is someone else in the house other than my family. It was never an option for us.

One other thing that I have to say that I got lucky with is not having a nightmare experience with an online service. Just recently, my personal trainer, Jenny, a mom of three kids, had a terrible incident with care.com. She hired a babysitter who turned out to be a fraud. Jenny had left her five-year-old and two-year-old with a sitter for a full-days' schedule of clients. She had a funny feeling; when she periodically checked her "nest" camera, her son was not in the crib at the right times. She called her sister-in-law to go and check on the kids, and her intuition was correct. The sitter appeared to be under the influence, and when Jenny arrived home, she found that her sister-in-law had called the police. The sitter was on prescription drugs and she was not who she said she was. The police checked her identification and ran a report on her. She had been arrested multiple times, once for child endangerment, and others for theft. Jenny's checkbook was in the sitter's purse and Jenny's clothing and other belongings were in grocery bags; the sitter was planning to steal them. Jenny did press charges and went to court, but the sitter never showed up. Now this is probably a rare story, but it happened. From then on, I felt that it was worth paying an agency to do the background checks, but also to hold them accountable. Nanny agencies hold their nannies accountable and help families like ours to stay safe but to also have great, reliable help.

To offer some more advice, I asked my mentor Dr. Cecile Yoon-Tarlie for her own input and experience.

Introducing Dr. Cecile Yoon-Tarlie

I graduated from my orthodontic residency program in 1998, and I began my career as a full-time associate and part-time clinical professor. Shortly thereafter I decided to venture on my own and open a startup practice. By the time my husband and I were ready to start a family, my start up practice was still in its infancy stages. The timing seemed perfect since I wasn't really too busy at the office and could afford the time to take adequate maternity leave as needed. I also lived less than a mile from my office, so if there were any true emergencies, I could pack up the baby and get to the office very quickly. Despite the apparent

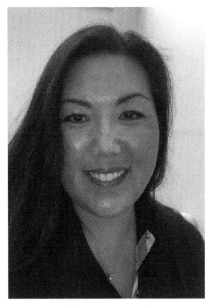

flexibility in planning for my leave, considering that it was my first pregnancy, this was preparation like no other. I needed to plan for my maternity leave, as well as office coverage for my staff and patients.

First, I had to decide whether I wanted a nanny or daycare. I quickly eliminated the daycare option because as a health care provider, it is commonly known that our schedules never end on time due to emergencies, unforeseen extended procedure times, patient consults, etc....and daycare centers are notoriously known for charging overtime for every second you are late. I knew I couldn't deal with that sort of stress, not to mention the increased likelihood of the baby catching some sort of illness or virus due to lots of children being in close quarters. And once your child is sick at daycare, you must pick up your child no matter what the time. This would have meant either canceling all the patients for the day (*not* an option) or finding a backup daycare and/or nanny, but *who*? As a solo practitioner, that was not an option for me, so I decided on a nanny.

Searching for a nanny was a new adventure for me. I started my due diligence about six months before my due date. I had to decide whether to look for a nanny by an agency or word of mouth. There are advantages and disadvantages to both. Looking at the cost factor alone, going with an agency can be expensive, but the benefit is that they do a lot of the leg work for you by checking references, doing background checks, initial interviewing, and sorting out candidates based on your requirements. Even if you decide on a candidate and it turns out that they are not quite right, you can still utilize their services until you find the right fit, with minimal or no extra charges. Word of mouth is much less expensive but can be time consuming, since you will have to do all the extensive leg work yourself, including background checks, reference checks, interviews etc. Well, I had six months, so I decided to try word of mouth first for a month, and if that failed, I would go to an agency. I asked friends, family, and even our subdivision's email chat group. I knew that I wanted a female, someone in her twenties or early thirties and with some experience. I did not want someone older who had a lot of experience because I wanted my nanny to follow my rules and guidelines for how I wanted my child changed, fed, napped, etc….no matter how crazy my rules seemed. I also wanted someone who drives and has a clean record. I also had a few other requirements as well regarding additional responsibilities—minimal housekeeping, menu planning, child activity planning, ability to be flexible in case I am running late due to patients, and someone with a safe car.

Through the chat group, I was able to narrow my list down to three candidates. I interviewed all three with my husband, and my mother was even there in the room with the baby. I gave an information sheet for them to fill out and had a list of questions. I took notes on the type of car they drove, what they wore, how good their English was, if they were prompt, if their nails were clean. I even allowed them to hold the baby, noting who washed their hands and who didn't. Fortunately, the nanny I was leaning towards previously worked at the local community center's child-care center, so I knew she already had a thorough background check; this saved me some time. Once I decided upon a nanny, I hired her under the pretense that there was a probationary period where she would be paid at the lower end of the pay scale that we negotiated, with the intent to increase her pay to the desired amount provided there was a very positive review and excellent continuation of care. This was all spelled out in the contract/agreement that we both signed. Given the various unpredictable end times of my day, I was sure to provide generous benefits. Our contract was renewed annually with a thorough review affecting her pay raise. By my third child, we moved out of state, and the town we moved to had a very reputable agency so I utilized the agency in finding our other nannies. It was costly but well worth every penny, especially being new to the area.

Now that my nanny situation was secured, I needed to next find coverage for my office. For my first child, as I mentioned earlier, my practice was in its early stages, so I was able to schedule my patients around my six-week maternity, with the plans to return for consults and patient starts about three or four weeks after delivery. I handled all the emergencies myself. During this maternity leave, the last three weeks were spent training my new nanny Monday through Friday while I was home, which also allowed me to leave the baby for one or two hours if I needed to go to the office.

For my second pregnancy, my practice was thankfully growing and I knew I really needed more adequate coverage in order to have patients progress in treatment. Luckily, I had recently joined an orthodontic disability group established by one of my local orthodontic instructors who was anticipating some time out of the office due to surgery. Our group consisted of approximately 10 orthodontists throughout the suburban area spanning three decades, so there were younger members like myself and more senior members as well. We had a legal document, which clearly defined the group's relationship with respect to what covering doctors were allowed to do, that there was to be *no* compensation, that all doctors would make every effort to participate, and more importantly, a code of ethics regarding not taking patients or staff away from the practice. Since this was my second c-section, I was eligible for coverage through my disability group. It was amazing and all the doctors were so kind and helpful. Many of the doctors covering my office enjoyed just checking out another practitioner's office and getting ideas. I highly recommend organizing a local one in your area if possible.

Despite *all* the months of thorough preparation, *nothing*—I repeat, *nothing*—can prepare you to be a mom. As most of us are probably your typical type-A, control-obsessed person, raising children is one of the most *unpredictable* jobs where chaos is the norm. We are not used to this…well, at least I wasn't, so I decided to start an interdisciplinary dental group focusing on educating our colleagues about the advances in each of our disciplines, and more importantly, providing support and understanding of being a new mom and a dental practitioner. This camaraderie of women was comprised entirely of female dentists of approximately at the same level within our career development (solo practitioners, group practitioners, and associates) and family development (we were either pregnant or had a little one at home) of all dental disciplines, preferably equal in specialty distribution where we would get together to discuss interdisciplinary cases we were treating, to have literature reviews, and more importantly, discuss our practices, businesses, and family life, namely *how to balance* it all. This sort of academic, business, and emotional support was amazing and therapeutic. Not only did we use each other as a dental resource, but also as a baby/family resource—which stroller to buy, which snacks are healthy, how to sleep train, who your pediatrician is, etc. At least having the needed support and resource proved to be very helpful, as we all navigated into motherhood together.

The best advice for other mommy dentists in business: *Don't* be afraid or embarrassed to ask for help, whether at home or at the office. Take care of *you* so that you can be the best in taking care of others.

Champaign as well as a bachelor of Dental Science (1993) while attending dental school at the University of Illinois at Chicago, College of Dentistry. She graduated (1995) with the highest of honors as a member of Omicron Kappa Upsilon (honorary dental fraternity). She received several awards including the American Student Dental Association Award for Excellence, The Pierre Fauchard Academy Award, The W. Howard Kubacki Award, The Dental Alumni Association Lifetime Award and the University of Illinois Alumni Association Leadership Award.

She continued with a post graduate orthodontic residency at the University of Illinois at Chicago, College of Dentistry and pursued a Masters in Oral Sciences. Her master's thesis won the Postdoctoral Poster clinical award in 1998 as well as invitations to present her research at the Moyer's pre-symposium at the University of Michigan and the Illinois Alumni Association Quadrennial meeting.

Her interests in leadership positions include serving as a delegate for the American Association of Women Dentists at an ADA invitational diversity forum, serving on the board of the Illinois society of Orthodontist as a trustee, Treasurer, Vice President and eventually the first female president of the state society. She was involved in the Dental Chicago Society Northside branch as a dinner chairperson, librarian,

---

treasurer, secretary, and vice president. At the national level, she served on the initial New and Younger Member advisory committee of the American Association of Orthodontists as well as its established council within the American Association of Orthodontists and as a delegate representing the Midwestern Society of Orthodontists. She even started her own all female interdisciplinary dental study club (LADE: Ladies advancing in Dental Excellence).

She continued her interests in academics working as a clinical assistant professor right out of residency, supervising residents and lecturing on growth and development. Her publications include articles in Seminars in Orthodontics, American Journal of Orthodontics and Dento-facial Orthopedics, and Women Dentistry Journal.

She has also been on local television shows and many panels discussing balancing a professional career, a leadership career and a family. Dr. Cecile Yoon-Tarlie recently moved to Massachusetts and plans to return back to work soon. She lives with her husband of more than 20 years and three children continually balancing her family's lives as well as finding time to enjoy working out, spinning, and organizing.

To connect with Dr. Yoon-Tarlie, contact her at MCTarlie@prodigy.net.

Chapter Eight
Don't Burn Bridges

Even though I live in a large city, the dental community is very small, especially in pediatric dentistry. The area that I practice in is very competitive and inundated with pediatric dentists. There are five pediatric dental offices within three miles of my office; yes, we are very saturated. Your reputation can make or break you, not just online, but among your peers as well. I was taught in dental school never to talk negatively about your colleagues, even the ones you have never met. I do believe in karma and that negativity can find its way back to you. We have all at one time or another seen a case done by someone else and thought that the work was subpar, but we shouldn't tell the patient that the work was terrible and blame the other dentist. We never know the circumstances and sometimes the patient is not always accurate in telling their dental history. I believe when those dentists speak poorly of others, it may have to do with their own insecurities, and they often make themselves look bad in front of the patient when they speak negatively of others. It's a sign of immaturity and poor judgment; just don't go there, and if you do know the other dentist, give a call and find out what happened, or get the scoop. We can't always win over every patient, and we have to remind ourselves that we are patients too, and we get along better with some doctors than with others.

In the city I live, many pediatric dentists practice orthodontics; in fact, many general dentists practice orthodontics. I, myself, have deep roots in orthodontics and started out in the orthodontic office at the age of 18. It was my part-time job during college and throughout dental school. I was even the assistant to the program director in the post-graduate department. I was thinking about going to orthodontic residency, but I felt a passion for pediatric dentistry and really wanted to learn more. I was burnt out working with niti wires, taking impressions, and placing bands, so I wanted to delve into pediatrics instead. I felt I could still practice orthodontics while being a pediatric dentist. Needless to say, it is still one of my passions, and I love treating phase-one patients.

I have a friendly competitor in the neighborhood who does not practice any orthodontics and refers everything to another office close by. Many of her patients end up in my office for a second opinion because the parent feels that the orthodontic office is not child-friendly. Often times, the patient does not add the name of their dentist because they feel embarrassed or uncomfortable telling me that they have come from the competitor's office. I have had several patients come in and start treatment with me, only to call back months down the line and say that their dentist is concerned about my work because they were told that "Dr. Yum is not an orthodontist."

I tell every parent before I start treatment that I am not an orthodontist, but this type of dentistry can be done by any dentist, depending on their training. One parent actually told me that she knew that the other dentist was trying to disparage me, but that she trusted me and that it was her choice as to where she wanted to take her kids for treatment. She then asked me not to say anything, as she didn't want any confrontation. I knew right away that I needed to contact the other doctor and try to smooth things over before this got out of hand. My colleagues were telling me to contact my lawyer to write a cease and desist letter, but my intuition was that I needed to be mature and reach out to try to smooth things over with her. After trying to reach her and calling and leaving messages, we were able to connect by email. I wrote, essentially, that since we were both part of the community, it was important to me to have a good relationship with her and to treat mutual patients with respect. She agreed with me on that and said that she wanted better communication from me as to what I was doing with "her" patients. I told her that most of them don't even mention her name or tell me that they don't want me to talk with her, but that, moving forward, if I knew the patient was coming from her office, I would write her a letter.

It finally came out what she was so upset about. It turned out that she was unhappy that her patients were coming back to her with sealants on their teeth. It is part of my practice that if my patients have appliances in their mouths, including fixed appliances and braces, I recommend dental sealants. I agreed that we—meaning any of my associates or I—will refer the patient back to her for sealants as long as we know she is the primary. When I think about the scenario, I can't help but think of what I would have done if the roles were reversed. I would have picked up the phone and had a mature adult conversation of my expectations and what I would have liked to see happen.

Open communication among peers is essential for professional relationships. There shouldn't be high-flying emotions or negative talk about another dentist in front of a patient, because at the end of the day, you make yourself look bad. You ruin your own reputation in front of the other dentist and most of all, your own patient. After 14 years of private practice, I had never had this kind of experience. As women and moms and business owners, I think it is so important to be supportive of one another, even if we are competitors. There is enough room in this space for all to run successful businesses. I've had orthodontics patients from other pediatric dental offices tell me that they want to switch over for hygiene; I tell them not to and speak highly of their dentists. Many parents tell me they think that it's very ethical of me not to have them switch over. The point is, I make it a point to speak highly of my colleagues, even though they are competitors.

Another relevant point about not burning any bridges has to do with your team members and co-workers. I learned through being a dental assistant that many assistants rotated around dental offices. I also learned that many of the associate doctors worked in several offices. To this day, I am still connected to co-workers that I met as dental assistants at the age of 18. One is a hygienist now, some are still assistants, and some have become dentists like myself. When I opened my second office in the suburbs, I received a resume via email. When I looked at the resume, I nearly fell off my chair and choked on my lunch because it was from a woman who was my friend's former office manager at her orthodontic office. Not only did I know her through my friend, this woman had worked the front desk at the office where I was a dental assistant at the age of 18. She had watched me blossom from sweeping the floors, pouring models, running errands, answering phones, filing charts, all the way to a practice owner. She had no idea that I was the owner of this office, and she submitted her resume online. She is my senior marketing coordinator of the office and has built her connections to general dentists from her previous role as office manager. Her connections and experience are invaluable to my practice. Had I not formed a good relationship with her during my days as a dental assistant, she may have not wanted to join me. We are a great team and I am blessed to have her.

In the same way, when I was an associate during my pediatric residency, I moonlighted at a pediatric dental office on Saturdays. That position turned into a part-time position when I finished, and I continued to work there for four years. While I was there, I learned that my relationships with my team were valuable. They were there to make my life easier, and since I had been an assistant, I could appreciate the work they were doing and I could give tips on how to make their lives easier. It was at that office that I formed a relationship with the office manager.

She and I had amazing ideas; we had a great relationship. It was as if we shared the same mind and often the same vision on how to make the office run efficiently. Our like-mindedness connected us in so many ways; it was refreshing to work with someone that could understand my needs as a dentist and execute the schedule accordingly. When I left to build my own practice, I wanted to take her with me, but my contract specifically stated that I was not to solicit employees of the office or the patients of the office. I hired a different manager and started without my favorite manager. After two years of opening my business, she reached out to me and wanted to join my team. I was very clear that a manager position was not available, but she didn't mind; she was just happy to join the team. Because we had such a great relationship those years I was an associate, she eventually came to work with me. In my career, I've come to realize that forming solid, healthy working relationships leads to connections and networking that are useful when hiring the right team.

An Interview with Dr. Beth Wylie

1. What does it mean in life to not burn bridges?

    To me, what it means to not burn bridges is to treat others with respect. You can disagree with people and have different opinions, and even need to distance yourself from another person, but it's how you do these things that will speak volumes about who you are. Visualize for a second the imagery of this. You burn that bridge to the ground, and you have no materials to rebuild it. You're just sitting there looking at it. And now it's not doing anyone any good at all.

2. Why is it important not to burn bridges both personally and professionally?

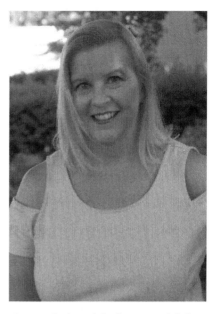

Why wouldn't it matter? Listen, what good does it do to burn a bridge? Once done, the chances of repairing a relationship are very low. The time, energy, and effort required to repair a broken relationship is a way higher cost than nurturing it to begin with. In business, that kind of damage can easily hurt your public reputation and will ultimately place your business at risk.

If you don't think that your personal life can and will affect your business life, let me assure you, you're mistaken. Acting out of anger or lashing out in hurt can easily cause more damage than can ever be repaired.

I don't want you to think that I would have you to give in to acting out of your values and integrity. Nothing should guide you more strongly than integrity, values, and faith. The catch is that we don't always agree on what the correct thing is. Respecting that someone disagrees with you is one of the most precious gifts we can share. Ending a business relationship is often necessary. Again, I stress it is *how* you end a relationship that matters far more than keeping a toxic one. Ending personal, toxic relationships is also necessary, but ending them in a manner that allows you to hold your head up the next time you see that person is far more valuable to you on a personal level. You have to be able to look at yourself in the mirror every day.

3. Have you ever burned a bridge and then regretted it?

Absolutely. I have taken great care in my business life, but I've made mistakes in my personal life that have cost me. Thoughtless comments made out of jealousy or anger, frustration or hurt feelings are the most damaging. We can only apologize afterwards, but spoken words of hurt can never be taken back. I have learned from personal experience that practicing kindness is always the best policy. If I've burned bridges professionally, they are just talking about me behind my back; I'm unaware of it.

4. Have you passed these lessons onto your children?

I pray I will. I've taught my kids, if nothing else, how to treat others. My daddy was one of the most genuinely kind people I ever knew. He was no one to be trifled with. He believed what he believed with passion, and his mind and position on a subject could very rarely be swayed, *but* he still listened with respect to others' opinions.

5. What advice do you have for another mommy dentist in business regarding this?

I think the most important thing we can do as moms and as humans is to remember to extend grace to others. If we judge someone only by our perception of their mistakes, we negate all the wonderful things about them. Yes, there are truly evil people out there; I believe that, but the majority of us are just trying to do the best we can every day. Isn't that what you are trying to do? I want people to look at the whole of my life, of who I am and who I'm trying to be and not just the portion where I screw it up. That's not the entire picture. And the whole picture of who I am is a person trying to make a difference in my community. I'm a mom desperately trying to raise good mini-humans. I'm a dentist trying to do my best for each and every little person who walks in my door. I'm a wife trying to live a happy life with my husband. And I'm a woman trying to be the best friend I can be to those in my circle, loving those I come into contact with. I don't have time to burn things down; I'm too busy trying to build them up. (And I love all of y'all!)

Dr. Beth Wylie is a native of Camden, South Carolina. She graduated with a B.A. in Psychology from Furman University and attended the Medical University of South Carolina in Charleston, where she received her Doctor of Medical Dentistry in 1996. She then specialized in pediatric dentistry, earning her certificate from Northwestern University School of Dentistry and Children's Memorial Hospital in Chicago, IL.

After her education, she began practicing in Sumter, South Carolina, where she's been in private practice at Carolina Children's Dentistry for 20 years as an associate and owner. Dr. Wylie is a proud member of the Junior Welfare League of Sumter, in the past serving as the Placement Chairman, and currently serving as the Assistant Secretary. She teaches Sunday School at Trinity United Methodist Church and has been married to Charlie for 25 years. Beth has two children, Holly and Jack, who she adores, and two dogs (Jet and Toby) and three cats (Muffin, Camden, and Malcolm). She is a swim and soccer mom, a reader, loves a good action film, and is a Disney fanatic. To connect with Dr. Wylie, please contact her at LWPoag@CCDSmail.com.

Chapter Nine
Location, Location, Location

One of the best pieces of advice my attending gave me, while I was a pediatric resident, was to live close to my office. At that time, since I was a resident, beggars couldn't be choosers, so I had no control over where I would live and where I would work. Once I started to work as an associate at a location about one hour away, however, the owner of that practice also told me to live close to where I worked. She owned an office in the suburbs, but she lived in the city and did the same commute. I watched her run her practice as a mom and she really needed everyone, including me, to help her with her practice and child. It wasn't easy to watch her drop everything and go and pick up her sick child at day care. It wasn't easy for me to drive one or two hours a day to work, when I could have been at the gym or meeting friends. So much time is lost in the car driving to and from work. That always stuck with me as an associate, and what my mentors relayed to me made more sense and would make even more sense as a mother.

Now that I have two toddlers at home and two businesses to run, it is essential to be close to them. I don't want to be stuck in a car driving for hours when I could be with them or doing something else. The commuting time is time that could be spent being more productive, so when I decided to open up my business, I wanted a location where I thought I could live. Choosing the location was a very important decision.

My dental career began when I was 18 years old, studying at Northwestern University. I had the opportunity to work at several dental offices while a student finding my way through life. It was because of my experiences that I began to draw upon how to find the best location. Once, I was a pediatric associate in a suburb and the owner was inside a bank on the second floor with no signage on the building. I thought, *How in the world is anyone supposed to find you if there is no signage?* In fact, the owner of the practice had built a space next door to where she was an associate for a general dentist. I don't know for sure if it would have mattered if the practice was located in a retail space on the ground floor, but I do think that it took a lot longer to build the practice. Another office that I had worked at had a great location, albeit, an hour, sometimes an hour-and-a-half drive for me. The office was in a busy strip mall at a busy intersection, which was very easy to get to. The mall had plenty of parking, restaurants, dry cleaners, nail salon, bank, and other retailers that brought people there. When I was seeing my patients, the parents would often drop off their kids and run errands. That was a big compliment to me that they would trust me enough to do that, but I really loved that I could fill my gas tank and go grocery shopping after my day was over. Not only was it cheaper in the suburbs, I could wait for rush-hour traffic to be done before going home. The only thing that was missing was a gym. I knew that one day I would own my very own practice and have associates working for me. In order to recruit in great talent, I knew that I would have to find locations that were easy to get to and have other amenities for other doctors to take advantage of. I know that location is crucial for the growth of the practice and to obtain and recruit great talent.

My flagship office in the city opened in 2009. It is my pride and joy; almost like having a child. I built it from scratch and still remember driving around town looking for the perfect location to start my dream office. It was a snowy February and my husband and I drove around in our truck looking at commercial spaces. We noticed a few businesses in the area that catered to kids, such as Gymboree and GapKids and decided that they could do the research and find premiere real estate. That night, we noticed a building under construction and it looked like commercial space on the first floor and residential above. We took down the number on the sign and called the next day. We were in luck! No one had rented the space out and it was a brand-new building. I was so excited that we found the perfect location. The rent was on the high side, considering the neighborhood we were in, but my window line, I considered to be my billboard. I considered my rent to be partly marketing because of my signage. The road is always backed with traffic and we receive phone calls from drivers that are stuck in traffic. I remember that when choosing my signage, I went with vinyl perforation so that I could see outside from inside but not the other way around unless it was dark outside. The signage was very kid-friendly and colorful; consistent with my branding. When we opened, I received phone calls from neighbors saying that my signage was obnoxious, but I didn't care. How else was I going to grab the attention of all the children in the cars or strollers? I also wanted to find a space near schools and a park. Lucky for me, I had four local schools a block away and a park opened up at the end of my block after my third year of being in business. Now, that was divine intervention and I was very grateful to God for all the blessings that came my way.

I rented the space for six years with hope to one day own the real estate. One day, I received a phone call from my landlord. He was ready to sell me the space—not just the 2300 square feet of mine, but also the 900 square feet next door, which was a hair salon. I was wondering why he wanted to sell at this time, so I went to visit my neighbor. It turned out that she wanted to close her business. I was going to have to rent out that space because I was not ready to extend my office yet. Luckily, I was able to find renters to take on a three-year lease.

When it became time to open up my second location, I knew that it was going to be a big endeavor. What drove me to do it was having 30 families move to the suburbs one summer, specifically to the north shore. This was actually a natural progression for families in the city. Most couples meet in the city or move here out of college, then they get married and have one or two kids and make it work until the kids need to go to school full time. Most families want to move to the suburbs to find a house with more space and a back yard and not have to pay a fortune. As I had more conversations about where they were going, I noticed that most were moving to Glenview, the area where I grew up. I thought, *Why am I losing these patient to the burbs? I worked so hard to get new patients and now I am losing them to the burbs?* Without taking on too much risk, I decided to rent an existing space two days a month to see if those patients would follow me. I worked on my days off and took two assistants with me, along with a laptop computer that had the software downloaded. I got the square to run credit card payments through my cell phone, or took payments by calling the city office to run the credit card number. Patients were staying with me and I could easily fill my day. It worked out because the office I rented was in Glenview and I could bring my kids to my parents' house for the day. It was a no-brainer that I open another scratch practice and that is exactly what I did. I found a store front in a strip mall down the street with everything I was looking for: Walgreens, Starbucks, Trader Joe's, and most importantly, Staples. Little did I know that the Good Will donation store two doors down from me brought 60 drop-offs a day. We began to have people walk in to book appointments. It has now been two-and-a-half years since we have opened, and about 6 months ago, the PetSmart opened next door; that was another blessing from God. People were starting to trickle in due to the new store next door. Again, location is so crucial to the marketing of your practice. Even if people aren't ready to make appointments or don't have kids themselves, they know that we are there because of all the other storefronts that are destinations. Even for my associates, they can actually work out at the gym next door or at Orange Theory across the street. They can fill up on gas on the corner or buy groceries at Trader Joe's. If we run out of paper, we can walk next door to Staples. Being in that shopping mall has been one of the best decisions for the business.

Because I had done the process before, I was able to recruit the same team and build another office in two months. During that time, I was pregnant with my son; he was born in August and the office opened that December. I took a six-week maternity leave and entrusted my office manager to make sure the office was exactly what we wanted. The timing was exactly what I had planned for. I knew that the growth would be slower in Glenview and I didn't need to be there often, but my husband and I were planning on moving to the burbs eventually once we didn't really need a nanny. I figured that we would move north once the office needed me more.

An Interview with Dr. Leslie Butler

1. How did you decide on where to open up your practices?

   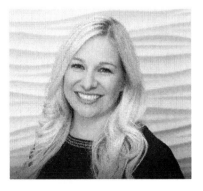

   I'm originally from Fullerton, CA. When looking to open a practice, I first thought, *Where do I want to raise my family?* A

81

new community? Near family? Near friends? What are the school districts and safety like in those areas? Once my husband and I talked, we decided to stay near family. This was a huge factor for us, as my husband's family lives in New Zealand. The only help we'd receive for our future children would be from my family. It also helped that I grew up in the area and knew many of the physicians and dentists in the community; my name was already known. Once we decided on Fullerton, CA as our new office's home, it came down to searching for just the right spot.

2. Was there anything in particular you were looking for in location? Did you have a list of requirements that you wanted in finding the perfect place?

Yes, absolutely! I needed a place for my fish tank. LOL! Honestly, I did; however, there were so many other important things that I was looking for as well. I had a vision and already knew what I wanted my office to look like and how I wanted it to feel. I wanted a minimum of 1700 square feet, I wanted a lot of windows, I needed to have extremely high ceilings (or the ability to raise the ceilings), and I honestly needed a place for my massive fish tank that I desperately wanted.

3. Is there such a thing as a perfect place?

Yes and No. I'm a huge believer of feeling or just knowing when something is right. I went through over 50 properties and potential spaces before I found it. I walked in and just knew within five minutes that this was the place for my office and I was going to fight for it.

4. What were the qualifiers in finding a location?

Community: where is it located? I wanted to be near downtown. It's an up and coming area and it's the only affordable location for young families to move into the community. Our city is highly sought after because of the *amazing* school district here; however, the average home price keeps a lot of younger families from purchasing a home here. Near downtown, there are smaller homes and two of the best schools in all of Southern California (an elementary and a high school), so I knew this is where I wanted to be.

Street: I wanted to be on a main street with good visibility and signage. We were able to find a building that had been completely renovated and even won awards for their landscaping. We're the corner unit facing the street, and we have lit-up street signage

Square footage: I needed a minimum of 1700 square feet or larger. I talked with many of my colleagues before this started and some regretted having smaller spaces. There is no place for them to go unless they move from their spaces entirely. The space I found was 2000 square feet, and I had a clause placed to have the first chance to rent the adjacent space if it was to become available.

Ceiling height: I took a contractor with me to all site visits. We opened the ceiling panels while there to make sure the ceilings could be raised to nine or ten feet. It was a deal breaker for me if they couldn't.

Fish tank: I needed to find an office where I could picture having the tank that I really wanted. The building also had to be able to support the weight of it if I was not on the first level.

Landlord: I wanted a reasonable and understanding landlord. This is something that can usually be determined in the first lease negotiation. The ones I chose were very easy to work with, willing to see things from my perspective, listened, and pretty much gave me everything I had requested, including money towards my build-out.

Rent: It has to be reasonable and realistic; if it isn't, your practice won't survive and you won't be able to afford your rent. I was able to successfully negotiate mine twice now, and with a small presentation each time, he agreed, both times to my terms.

Utilities: I wanted a space where my utilities were included. As a dentist, our electric and water bills have the potential of being extremely high. Finding a location where all my utilities were also included is a huge benefit to me now, and especially when I was a start-up practice.

Parking: Is there enough parking for your office? This is *always* a problem. We have underground parking for our team members, and our patients park on the main level; however, parking on the street is near impossible because we are only two blocks away from our local community college and our street is the first block of unrestricted street parking. I wish we had looked at this more closely. Sometimes it's a huge problem for us and our patients.

Other tenants in the building: Are they going to be nice and friendly? Are there other doctors/dentists in your building? We only have a chiropractor in our building, and then 50% of the building is rented by a Foster/Therapy/Adoption agency that is amazing. They have all been great neighbors.

5. How important is it to live near where your offices are located?

Very; especially now that I have two children. It's easy to get to work (less than 15 minutes) and easy to get home. I can run to my kids' school on lunch if I want to stop by or if there is a problem. I used to commute one to three hours each way before I had kids, even when I was pregnant with my daughter. It wasn't a big deal then. Now, I still work in one location that has me driving one to two hours each way, and I *hate* those days. The only thing keeping me there is the money; otherwise I'd leave in a heartbeat. It puts so much stress on me, and I hardly see my kids at all the day of the week I work there. That is very hard for me.

6. Do you have any advice for MDIBs, as to what has made it work for you?

Support! I have an amazing family and team around me. My husband and parents have been my #1 cheerleaders. If I need help, they are always the first to jump in. From running a million errands for the buildout/design process to coming in and helping sort mail. Anything I need, they are there. As for my team, I have an awesome team of professionals behind me as well. From my attorney, CPA, and financial planner to my contractors and dental representatives, they have all made this process so much easier for me than it could have been.

7. Is it worth paying more rent for the right place?

No, I personally don't think so. There will always be the right spot, but it just may take some extra time to find it. It's not worth struggling and working your tushy off to just pay the rent. None of us should live like that. There is the saying, "Don't live house poor." I feel the same way with regards to your practice rent. It may look perfect and beautiful on the outside, but that one little thing can make you regret the decision forever.

8. How important is it to you to own the real estate?

Very. It's on the horizon for us, but not quite reachable yet. *That* is what is going to secure your future and your retirement, not your practice. You can't ever consider the sale of your practice retirement, because you never know what could happen to you or the business. Real estate is a safer, long-term investment, however. We have already reached out to our building owner and will start negotiations in the next couple of years to purchase our building with a couple other investors. It's our long-term retirement plan.

Dr. Leslie Butler is a Pediatric Dental Specialist who grew up in Orange County, California. She has worked in a Pediatric Dental practice in Newport Beach for 10 years, but then decided to open her own practice, Butler Pediatric Dentistry, in Fullerton, CA, in 2013. Dr Butler and her practice have become the leading Pediatric Dental practice in Orange County serving patients of all ages with Autism Spectrum Disorders. She is opening her second practice in Villa Park, CA called Villa Park Pediatric Dentistry. She received her Bachelor of Science in Biology from Azusa Pacific University, with minors in Chemistry and Biblical Studies. She has actively participated in many community-based and international dental mission programs for children where she developed her love for children's dentistry.

After taking a year off from school and working as a dental assistant in Berkeley, CA, Dr Butler received her D.D.S. from Loma Linda University, and then completed her 2-year specialized Pediatric Dental training and Master of Science in Dentistry degree at Loma Linda University Medical Center. Her two-years of Pediatric specialty training prepared her to work with children with special needs and focus on dental

---

disease prevention. During her residency program, she also co-led a dental mission trip to the Galapagos Islands.

Over the many years of practicing, Dr Butler has found her love and passion not just for her patients and profession, but also for the business side of Dentistry. When not practicing dentistry and running her two practices, Dr. Butler enjoys spending time with her husband, and two young children. She enjoys going to the movies, reading a great book, spending time at Disneyland, and photography. Traveling continues to be one of her greatest passions and looks forward to leading more dental mission trips to different corners of the world.

To connect with Dr. Butler, please reach out to her at www.ButlerPediatricDentistry.com.

Chapter Ten
Not Enough Hours in a Day

As working moms, I think we all agree that there are not enough hours in the day. I often think to myself, *What in the world did I do with all that time I had before I had kids and a business?!* I wish that I could have two hours more to get more sleep, or read that book, or just talk on the phone and catch up with friends and family. We get behind in writing our chart notes and behind in doing things for the office. In my family, I am the social secretary for me and my husband, so it's hard to make plans and fill our calendars with dinners with friends. Now that my kids are getting older, their schedules are more challenging to fill than mine. How do we do it? How do we really do it all and get everything we want out of our lives? For me, I have really had to prioritize what I need and want in my life and I don't sweat the small stuff. And again—I stress—find an assistant to help you get organized.

One way to really stay organized is to get a calendar, whether it is online or written down old school, it is much better to have everything written down in order to keep all things organized. Often times, I calendar all my events and I still manage to screw it up! Since I still work on some Saturdays, my husband is on birthday duty and takes our kids to their classmate's parties. I have sent him to the wrong place at the right time and to the right place at the wrong time. I have gone to my trainer on the right day at the wrong time and I have gone to a doctor's appointment on the wrong day at the right time. No matter how organized I am and have pop-up reminders on my phone, I still get it wrong. There is only so much I can handle, and if all my brain power gets used up at work and on my kids, I allow myself to make some mistakes. When any of my patients come to my office and think they have an appointment and it's really for another date and time, I am more than understanding and will fit them in since they are already at the office. The one pet peeve I have is when doctors' offices don't accommodate me if I come at the wrong time. Sure, I get it; they are busy just as I am and they don't need to take me, but if I am already there at the office, is it really that hard to take me? Please cut me some slack; I will definitely cut you some slack!

Now, what about exercise? Before I had children, I lived at the gym and couldn't go without one day of working out. I had a great schedule that I could abide by and I was addicted to working out every day after seeing patients. I even ran a half marathon without training for it because I was in such great condition. Even after I built my practice, I made sure to work out and had a trainer come to my office or to my house if I could not make it to the gym. I continued practicing yoga during my maternity, but once my first child came, I had less and less time to work out. I tried to exercise three times a week, but then the guilt of not spending enough time with my daughter would set in. When the second office opened and I had my second child, it was even harder to find time to exercise. Even if I could find the time, I was too exhausted at the end of the day to even get on the treadmill. I guess my kids are still young and still wake up in the middle of the night and keep me up, and again, when my spouse is out of town for work, I'm the one that has to stay up in the middle of the night. That actually takes a toll on your body because you are not receiving continuous sleep. I do try to practice yoga once a week at my office. My instructor comes to me during my lunch hour and I try to meditate in the middle of the day. That is a hard thing to do, though, because it is hard to turn off my brain and focus. I do know of many moms that have workout equipment at their offices and just workout at the office, but I find that hard to do in the middle of the day. Those last five pounds are just the hardest and you can't just use baby weight as an excuse when you had him three years ago. Needless to say, I'm still trying to find out when the best time is to make it happen. Many moms will squeeze it in before their kids wake up and many work out at their office at lunch and many workout at night. I try to fit it in when I can, but like my friend, Jenny Sloan says, make an appointment with a trainer. It's like making a dentist appointment.

It would be so nice to have the time to cook again. Ah, the life I had before I had kids, where I had so much time I don't remember what I did with it. I do vaguely remember having a recipe box and loving to cook. I would watch cooking shows while working out on a machine and try to recreate recipes at home. All the gorgeous wedding gifts that we had received were put to good use; the china, the pots and pans, the wine glasses. And now, half the time I don't even know where they are in my kitchen. Embarrassingly, we had a fancy, red KitchenAid mixer given to us, and I just used it for the first time to make cookies with my kids, only nine years later. Thank goodness it still worked and thank God for YouTube. I'm not one to read manuals, so I tend to YouTube everything if I'm not sure how to do something. I even pull up YouTube to show my patients what expanders look like and how they work.

Some of my colleagues hire a chef and some have nannies that cook for them. I am lucky to have a nanny that enjoys cooking for us, but for those that don't there are meal delivery programs that seem to work well. My friends swear by the instant pot and I have yet to try it, but it does look great. One of these days, I will go back to cooking.

Introducing Dr. Linty John-Varghese

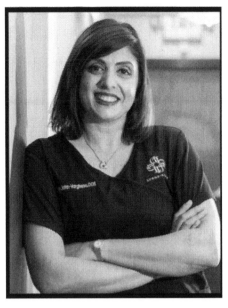

Isn't that everyone's problem?! I'm convinced that time is a rigged concept where we get to *think* we have 24 hours, but clearly, it's a very well-thought-out conspiracy by some man in his nineties who had the last laugh. Well, I'm onto you, old gone man! How many times have I thought I still have time to do those three things that I planned all day, and I look at my cell phone, it's 9:30pm. Now to divulge an observation that seems like aliens control my body; when I look at the time, my eyelids lose their strength and simply gets lead-heavy because of some digits on a tiny electronic face that inevitably dictates my hypothalamus to start shutting down like the computer; and my kids are still not in bed for some insane reason. At this very time, my husband has once again disappeared into a black hole in my home that I still can't ever find; very similar to the black hole that my assistants go into when I look for them in my tiny practice. Finally, with my kids tucked in bed, my brain has opted to go into zombie mode. I look at the mirror while brushing my teeth, and looking back at me is someone else's haggard face still wearing black scrubs, because who has time to change or comb their hair while running around with kids for their activities or working on their projects?!

See?! *Conspiracy!* Who stole my time?!

From the time I wake up to get ready, check on my kids, run to work, race against time seeing patients who clearly think that they are the only person that I see all day, while secretly scouting my staff to see if they're doing their job, running after lab work that hasn't returned yet, making sure that bills are collected for my back breaking labor despite my incessant love for my profession, and the dumb ideas I have to give my work away for free time and time again in the desperate attempt to be liked and not to offend the patient, while completely discounting that insurance companies are eating at my hand one finger at a time. Am I the only one who does that?

Oh, wait! Why didn't they pick that call? What?! Is that patient upset? Make it right, people! We can't have a bad review on social media. Kiss their behind! Ouch!

My shoulders hurt again! Why is that overhead light shining on my patient's chest instead of their teeth? Hmm...why don't I invent a seeker on the overhead light to find the mouth? *Suction*! Patient is drowning here! Squirrel... Poof! Gone. What was I talking about? Amid my ongoing crazy day, my head reels with ideas, like I'm in the tenth dimension of string theory, no one capturing my genius on paper, or inventing them for that matter. Am I really here, or is this the tenth D? Why am I not in Beverly Hills, living in Air; Bel Air—lounging by the pool, crisping my brown to toast, while a 20-year-old Fabio brings me my cucumber-infused water in a tall, chilled Versace glass. Wow! I must have slept with my eyes open while brushing my teeth again.

Dentistry—ahh, now that is a passion that never ends for me. Being a self-proclaimed CE junkie and professional student, it only means that I have so much exploding junk in my head that my hygienist hates calling me for an exam because, between my emotionally connected story of some sort and my elaborate, never-ending exam, along with repeating everything they just said 20 minutes ago to the patient, I truly feel that 60-minute hygiene appointment is not fair on me. I wish an hour had 90 minutes; I have so much to say.

Besides that quirk, I have the innate need to humanize teeth. They are all my 28, sometimes 32, and sometimes less than 10 dear friends. I look into the oral abyss and get lost in the stories that they tell me. It's a puzzle; it's a mystery. I feel like James Sully in *Avatar*, traveling into the Navi world to learn the secrets of the Oral Cavitaria, to represent them and the need to advocate for them.

My patients are just as nerve-wrecked as everyone in a dental chair, as they like to believe that my purpose in life is to inflict pain on poor defenseless beings; such is the stigma of our profession. My challenge is to change their belief in the system and to let them know I've got them and will keep them safe.

Then a show it is; if I can empathize yet humor them throughout the procedure, the response is outstanding. They forgive me for the injection that they detest, as I can understand; who really wants to be poked by a needle? And then there is the dreaded drill—why can't the drill play music instead, like the kid's electric toothbrush? Is that too much to ask for, dental world? Wait! That's a great idea! Maybe I should incorporate a Bluetooth chip in every handpiece to add music and convert the drill hum into that of music. Now, how do I do that? When am I supposed to work on that? I'm already running behind. Hey, but my patients love me. Or so I think...

I do have to admit I have high energy and spunk, despite how lousy a day can be. I empower my staff to be responsible for my patients like they made everything happen. It's funny, but when you transfer power, suddenly, they believe that the patient is there because of them. It's a big game changer in my practice because it's never my practice; it's *our* practice, and they are *your* patients, who trust you. I am but a guest. The practice becomes less about me and more about each staff member, and ultimately,

I do get a winning team who think they are all non-DDS dentists. Well, I know it's not ideal, but it works for me. Now, I want more...

I want to think outside the box. Ideas are genius. I like to believe time is a well-orchestrated idea between the sun and Earth. Therefore, time is genius, yet someone steals my time. I want to say it's called excuses, being lazy, not maximizing, being inefficient. Is that true?

Maybe I can figure out how to do it, but then again, who has the time? I listen to a lot of motivational speakers, and they say that if it's not on the schedule, it does not happen. Let me tell you that exercise has been on my schedule every day for the past few months. Ask me how many times that actually happens. I literally do a million other things just to sabotage my scheduled exercise time. I clearly proved some successful speaker wrong. I should be a *speaker*. Yes, that's it! That's only thing missing in my life, along with the multiple things I promise myself that I will get to.

I've realized that things only get done if you really want it to happen. I guess I know the answer to that one.

I work like a mad woman, I have a loving, supportive family whom I do enjoy torturing, I have limited social affairs by choice, but I'm still not fulfilled. My mind wants more out of life. Sometimes I think I have a severe case of FOMO. Missed time is missed opportunity, and neither are coming back. It dawns on me, and yet when life goes rolling by, following the same rhythmic, daily rituals, and my ideas and thoughts get subdued by them, and they are gone. I wish I wrote them down, I wish I knew how to act on my thoughts, I wish I knew how to make them happen, but who has the time for thoughts and ideas? That's for Disney to do, but then how does Disney make it happen?

As my mind wanders, I want to fly with the Eagles, I want to go to Mars strapped in next to Elan Musk on SpaceX, I want to collaborate with Jeff Bezos before we become United States of Amazon, I want to know how every great mind works, I want a team of inventors creating every idea that constantly sparks in my head, and let me tell you, my head is flooded with random great ideas and their tangents, none of which will ever materialize because who has the time? To the grave with me, it will go.

But *wait*! This isn't the end. Sleep is overrated. There will never be enough time if that's all I concentrate on. I have to train my mind to conquer, to overcome my weakness, to schedule better, to make time for myself, to seek out masterminds geared towards changing the world, to stop making excuses for my shortcomings. It isn't easy.

I am not perfect, but I am *not done*.

Dr. Linty John-Varghese took a multi-national route to her private practice in Dayton, Ohio. Starting life in Dubai, she initiated her career with a Bachelors in Dental Surgery in India, followed by DDS with Honors in Implants from NYU, a GPR at the VA in Dayton, OH, and then worked at the Wright Patterson Air Force Base as Contract Dentist, where she enhanced her dental knowledge during interactions with some powerful minds of the specialists there.

Four years later, she bought an existing successful private practice, invested further to become an avid CE learner, changed the practice to exclusively Restorative and Cosmetic Dentistry, tripled the revenue of an already lucrative practice, and finally started to transition from a PPO practice to FFS, all in a six-year span to date. Filled with positivity for her profession, she now gives back to the community by mentoring college students with interests in dentistry. She is passionate about motivating dentists, and also works in collaboration with 'Mastery Lab' to coach dentists by empowering them to move forward towards their goals, by trusting their need to succeed, by allowing for change in their mindset, and by letting go of their own limiting beliefs.

With three kids in school whom she loves to challenge, and a spouse who supports her incessant fire, she lives by one line, 'Don't aspire to make a living; aspire to make a difference!'. If you ever have a fleeting moment of self-doubt or dejection, please reach out to her at LintyJohn@hotmail.com. She will be happy to guide you through it.

Chapter Eleven
How Much is Your Time Worth?

This part of the book stems off of not having enough hours in a day, but focuses instead on time management and how an hour of your day is really important because of how valued your time is. An hour is an hour. I learned this lesson at the age of 16 when I was in my junior year of high school. I wanted to have a part time job so badly, but my parents were against it. Being Korean-American, my parents wanted me to be the model student and basically stay home and study all day, but there was something in me that really wanted to be in the real world and gain experience before venturing off to college. I heard that there were some students that were on the pre-medical track in their senior years that worked at my pediatrician's office part time after school and on Saturdays. I asked about the position and my friend, Nancy, who worked at the office filled me in and told me to come and interview. It was my very first time in an official job interview, so I was a bit nervous. The funny thing was that it was my very own pediatrician that I was meeting with. He didn't really ask me that many questions and since he knew my parents really well, he just gave me the job. Nancy showed me the ropes and the basics of what my job entailed. I was getting paid seven dollars an hour to do the basics. Eventually, the good doctor over time increased my wages to $11 an hour. I was interested in going to medical school while in high school, but one day I was faced with tragedy. A baby had died at the hospital and I remember the grief that family and the doctor faced when it happened. I just couldn't bear the thought of dealing with life and death. It was during that time that I also had to study for college entrance exams and my parents hired a private tutor to help me prepare. My tutor came to my house and was paid $40 an hour for the time I met with him. My father made me pay him myself and I didn't understand what the purpose was for that. One day I asked my dad, "Dad, why don't you pay him, why do you make me pay the tutor?" My father smiled and he sat me down and asked, "Grace, how much do you make at the doctor's office in one hour?" I said, "I make $11 an hour." Then he said, "How much do you pay the tutor for one hour?" I replied, "Well, I guess you give me $40 to give him for that hour." "Okay, then. When you work at the doctor's office, how much money does he make in one hour?" "Hmmmm…well, sometimes he makes $100, but then he sees patients every 15 minutes and sometimes he makes $200 in 15 minutes." At that moment, the lightbulb went on and I had an a-ha moment. The lesson he was teaching me is that an hour of time has value to it. The value depends on your job and what career you have, and he was teaching me that the level of education has an association to your compensation. For a high school student, you make less than that of a teacher who also makes less than someone with a medical degree. It was a very important lesson for me because it drove me to study harder and to pursue an education.

This lesson also pertains to our professional lives. Often, dentists don't place value on his or her work. You hear of so many dentists writing off balances or writing off emergency visits for their patients because they feel badly about charging. I used to do the same thing when I was an associate because I wanted to help people and wanted to be the nice guy, but as I gained more experience and gained more insight, I learned that it's ok to charge patients for emergencies and other procedures. I remember working as an associate when my office manager asked why I was not charging the patient after an emergency procedure. I said that I was happy to help out and the procedure was a simple extraction. She then sat me down and asked me a few questions.

1. Did you use any anesthetic?
2. Did you have an assistant help you?
3. Did you use any other supplies, like disposable bibs?
4. Did you spend at least 15 minutes in the room?

Well, of course, all my answers were yes. She proceeded with, "Well, are you going to pay for all of that yourself?" I asked her what she meant and she responded with, "Who is going to pay for the anesthetic, the assistant's time, and all the other supplies?"

Again, I had another a-h" moment and quickly realized that someone was going to have to pay for all of that, and this time it was the owner of the practice, but she told me that moving forward, if I was going to hand out free dentistry, it was going to come out of my own pocket. I can tell you that I quickly stopped treating patients for free.

I think that we, as dentists, are very giving and caring people. We genuinely want to help others and so it is a natural inclination to offer our services at no charge, but where we then get hurt is when those patients don't appreciate our time and services, or when the business suffers because we are not making enough money to operate the business. We have to remember that our time is well deserving of compensation. We have loans to pay, we have businesses to run, we have mouths to feed. Please remember to pay yourself and choose your charities wisely; don't let them choose you.

Introducing Dr. Sharhonda Lewis

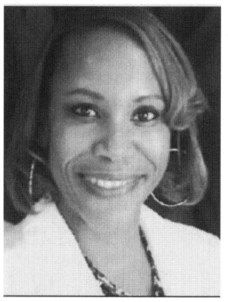

The journey to practice ownership began for me in November 2006. Never in a million years did I think I would become owner until I was approached by my former employer who decided to sell the practice. I figured it was an opportunity that I could not pass on, so I decided to venture into entrepreneurship.

As the years passed, I cannot say that it's been easier; I would rather say that I have to choose which situations I will allow myself to ponder over and which ones I'll just choose a quick solution for and move on. Being an African American woman and a mother has its own challenges in itself, but adding business owner of a dental practice to my many other titles just adds to the chaos that goes on in my world each and every day. The reason I say the word challenging is because a majority of the population tends to pull on a woman's emotions more than it does males. In the beginning of my road to owning a business, I have encountered patients who would break down in tears because of either not being able to financially afford their necessary dental treatment, or they were going through a personal situation in their life and simply needed someone to talk to. Since I have a family practice, I tend to form relationships with my patients. If they are regulars, in a sense, I end up knowing the entire family. From that family, they will refer their friends and other family members to me. I feel extremely grateful that someone will refer a loved one to me for their dental care, but along with some of those referrals, certain people will attempt to pull on your heart strings a little just to get a lower price. It became such a trend, especially with me that I decided to reach out to a male dental school classmate who owns an Orthodontic practice. One statement I will never forget from him is when he told me, "Women business owners tend to make decisions based off of emotions." What I took from our conversation is that in order to run a successful business, an owner has to possess the power of discernment. As women, we have to decide what is the truth and do what is best for us and our loved ones, especially as a mom. Our families depend on the finances of our business. For me, once my children came into the equation, finances are important because that is how I provide for them.

As women entrepreneurs *we have to know and realize our worth.* People will buy what they want and beg for what they need. Medical and dental care should not be negotiable. The field of dentistry is swamped with providers that negotiate fees with patients. Just think, if we all stuck to our fees and did not discuss the possibility of a lower price at the practice down the street or around the corner, how successful would we all be? This haggling attitude is the reason a majority of the population shops around for their dental needs. In my experience, medical practices do not have this type of behavior. Also, patients that need certain medical procedures performed are not asking their physician what the cost is for a particular treatment. As a profession, we all need to *stop* this behavior. Dental patients know they can go around the corner and possibly get certain treatment performed at a cheaper cost. This problem is not just a female business owner issue, but it involves male owners as well. If we stop this poor behavior, the dental profession would be respected more.

Dr. Sharhonda Washington was born in Houston, TX. As early as the age of five, she dreamed of becoming a doctor. She continued to thrive in academics throughout high school. After taking one visit to Xavier University of Louisiana during her senior year in high school, she knew this was the university for her.

After graduation, she became a student at Xavier University of Louisiana, majoring in Biology Pre-Med. In May 1996, she graduated from Xavier and couldn't decide in which sector of medicine she wanted to concentrate, so she moved back to Houston and began teaching 7th and 8th grade science in a middle school. After two years of teaching, she decided that it was time to concentrate on her dream once again. A college friend, also a dental student, encouraged her to attend dental school. Later that year she was accepted and decided to attend Meharry Medical College School of Dentistry in Nashville. After graduation, she attended a General Practice Residency at the Veterans Administration Hospital in Houston. Once that one-year program ended, Dr. Washington worked at a community health care center in Wichita Falls, Texas for almost two years. After that assignment ended, she moved back to Houston and started work as an associate at a private practice, which she now owns today.

Dr. Washington is now the owner of Allday Dental Associates in Houston, which provides an array of dental services including orthodontics and cosmetic dentistry. She has taken multiple continuing education courses in orthodontics for adult and pediatric patients. This service has greatly expanded her practice to provide more options for her patients. During her down time, she enjoys spending time with her family and is an avid basketball, cheer, and dance mom. She is also involved in her church and community activities, which include educating others on the importance of oral health.

Dr. Washington's favorite quote is by Dr Martin Luther King, Jr. "The ultimate measure of a man is not where he stands in moments of comfort or convenience, but where he stands in times of challenge and controversy." To connect with her, please email her at DrSWashington@AlldayDental.com.

Chapter Twelve
Giving Back

When I was a dental student, I remember one of my first lectures, and the doctor who was giving the lecture welcomed us with a reminder that being in healthcare was to serve our patients. With that service came an attitude of giving back to the community. He impressed on us that dentistry was about helping people and improving lives and not just about making money.

That lecture has stayed with me for over 15 years. Every day, we are faced with opportunities to give, whether it is to visit schools and educate young kids about dental health, to volunteer at a clinic, or even to go on a mission trip to help those in need. Every day I receive a letter in the mail to support schools, religious organizations, and local businesses, but what really sticks with me is the opportunity to serve where my heart is. It is not easy to decide which organizations to support because I only have limited funds, but it's about where there is need and where I feel that I can contribute the most.

Every February is National Children's Dental Health Month and as pediatric dentists, we often go out and educate kids on dentistry and the importance of having a healthy mouth and on health in general. The teachers love it and the kids enjoy it. This is a time where we spend a lot of our time out of the office and in these schools. We sacrifice seeing patients and making money in order to give back to our community and to these children.

Another opportunity to give back is to go on dental/medical mission trips with different organizations or through religious organizations. I once had an opportunity to go to an orphanage in Mexico to help treat the kids and adults. It was a wonderful way to see how these children lived in a very clean and happy environment. They were well taken care of and they were of all ages with adults everywhere to supervise. It almost seemed like a summer camp because it was run so well, but once we left the camp and actually visited with families that were impoverished, that was where I felt compelled to help. These were families that didn't have any help and could not enter the orphanage. It seemed to me so backward because the kids with parents were the ones that really needed clothing and medical attention and the children that were in the orphanage were well taken care of through all the supporting organizations. It makes you count your blessings when you are so far removed from your own home and country; it makes you realize the blessings you have. Helping others in need not only helps them; it really helps you.

As my profile grew in my city where I practice, my patients and friends invited me and my husband to many of their charities and organizations. We often attended many galas and banquets and offered our monetary donations.

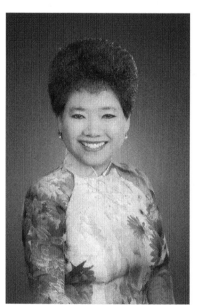

Introducing
Dr. Emily Letran

I was born during the Vietnam War in the late 1960's. When I was 7, the war ended and the Communists took over the country. A year after that, my mom passed away due to cancer.

I grew up with extended family: my father; my two aunts (his younger sisters), and my five siblings and cousins.

As a teenager, I remember living a life of scarcity. I used to stand in line at the government stores to buy food for the family. My aunt would bake a single plain cake with no frosting to celebrate our group birthday once a year. Every week, the electricity would be shut off in the neighborhood for a whole day. I would sit out in the balcony, holding up my notebook, using the lights from the soccer stadium close by to study.

Six years after the Communists took over, the government started drafting all the young men to go to war against the Chinese in the North and the Cambodians in the West. At this point, my aunt decided to leave the country, taking my brother and four other cousins to avoid the draft. I remember, as if it were yesterday, my dad telling me, "You're the oldest girl in the family. You need to go help your aunt," and sending me on my way. At 13 years old, saying good bye to my father, standing by a small bridge in the countryside, I never knew that was the last time I would ever see him. That same night, my aunt and the six of us kids, ages seven to 16, escaped on a fishing boat to find freedom. We were on the ocean for seven days and arrived at the refugee camp in Malaysia.

Three and a half months of living in the refugee camp really taught me a lot about humanity. I heard horror stories of boat people who got raped, robbed, kidnapped by pirates, or died at sea. I met young kids who survived their journeys without parents. I learned to receive, give, and share everything in the camp. I remember waiting around after each English class to pick up morsels of chalk, so I could write vocabulary words multiple times on the wall to learn the language. By the time we left the refugee camp, my heart was full of gratitude. I was grateful my family was together (my aunt, my brother, and four cousins), that we had a chance to learn English, and that we received food and fresh water every day. I told myself that when I had a chance, I would need to give, to help others around me.

Imagine coming to a foreign country without your parents and not knowing the language. I used to go to school with a pocket dictionary, and at home we had the biggest version of the English-Vietnamese Dictionary to help us study. There were 10 people sharing a two-bedroom apartment, so I slept on the floor for several years. The only table we had was the dining table. Sometimes I just sat on the floor, flipping a cardboard box as my table for studying. We received government aid during those years, including free lunches at school. At the age of 13, I went from living with my father to being a refugee, and then to a kid in America with opportunities. I felt grateful because I was a survivor. I also felt obligated to live life to its fullest potential because of the sacrifice my father had made for me.

After three years of undergraduate work and four years of dental school, I was eager to go out and make a difference. I quickly learned that even as a new associate with not much to show (no experience, no assets, no reputation), I was better off than a lot of people. The patients in the medical clinics reminded me of my past, and I treated them with respect. When the patients could not speak English well, I tried my broken Spanish to put them at ease. I made giving my way of life, whether it was to give respect, empathy, or financial resources.

Several years ago, the mother of one of my patients shared with my staff that she was really struggling to make the monthly payment for braces and saving up money to send her son to a band competition out of state. Without hesitation, I gave the mother a check for $1000. I know it was more than what was needed. I wanted to help more than just one kid go to the competition. I understood the sacrifice of a parent and the opportunity of a lifetime for the teenager. Another one of my patients shared with us that her house burned down. I immediately sent out an email to all my patients asking them to donate money, and that I would match every dollar they gave. We raised a good amount of funds, and the patient was surprised to receive the gift from our dental offices.

My biggest inspiration to give back came from learning the story of a dentist in Florida who provided free dental care in his community. He created a national movement. I started with two days of free dentistry a year, one in each of my offices, then quickly moved on to monthly free dentistry day, operating my non-profit organization, www.SmileChampions.org. On those days, we provide basic dental care for veterans and families with a disadvantaged background. I have never forgotten that one of those patients drove 100 miles to be the first one in line at 5am for free dentistry day. A few months later, after he got a job and insurance, he came back to the office and invested several thousand dollars in his smile. Sometimes people just need a little help to start their journey.

I believe *giving* is a way of life. My patients don't just appreciate what I do for them as patients, such as movie nights, patient appreciation dinners, and you-are-the-hearts-of-our-practice day. They love what I do as part of the community, providing free oral cancer screenings, educating about sleep apnea, donating to summer reading programs, and constantly creating social impact.

One of my goals in life is to become a world-famous philanthropist because I had seen what one can achieve by helping others and having a servant's heart. With the right association and positioning, I will be able to influence others to do the same thing: spreading love and positive impact right where you are and with what you have. I believe as a High-Performance Coach, I can effectively achieve this goal to reach out to many professionals and inspire them to do what I do, so our practices can all operate with the same mission to change lives through *giving*.

Winston Churchill said, "We make a living by what we get, but we make a life by what we give." I hope I inspire you by what I have shared and will see you alongside my journey, making a difference in people's lives with a servant's heart.

Dr. Emily Letran is a general dentist who owns two multi-specialty group practices in Southern California. She received her Bachelor of Science in Biology from UC Riverside (magna cum laude, Phi Beta Kappa) in three years. She is a graduate of UCLA School of Dentistry (Dean's Apollonian Scholarship) and received her Master of Science in Oral Biology from UCLA at the same time in four years. After graduation, she participated in the General Practice Residency at Loma Linda VA Medical Center in Loma Linda, CA. and a mini-residency at Rancho Los Amigos Medical Center in Downey, CA., where she attained additional training in treating geriatric and medically compromised patients.

As a mother of three, Dr. Letran creatively balances work, family life, after-school life and her personal life as a growing entrepreneur. She continuously takes courses in clinical dentistry, practice management and marketing, attending multiple business forums to improve her skills to better serve patients. Her favorite activities include reading, creative writing, and "hanging out" with her three children - whether playing tennis, watching Netflix, or enjoying Starbucks together.

You can connect with her at www.DrEmilyLetran.com or emily@exceptionalleverage.com.

Chapter Thirteen
It Takes a Village

People often ask me, "Where do you find the time," and "Do you ever sleep?" I often laugh and share my secrets of how I can get so much done in a short amount of time. I've learned to surround myself with a village. I have a village in my home and I have a village in my office. Creating a village, in my mind, means surrounding myself with people that love me, that root for me, and that share my vision. How do you find your village? How do you know who is rooting for you? If I didn't have a village, I wouldn't be able to do all the things I want. The dishes and the laundry—I don't do those things, so that I can spend time with my kids and do my work and all the things I want to do.

Who's in my village? Those people would be my beloved family; my parents, who live close enough to drive and pick my kids up and take them to lessons and activities; my nanny, who is my house keeper and second mom to my children; all of my part time babysitters, who can watch my kids after I put them down so that I can go out with my husband for date nights and nights for me to go and get a quick manicure and pedicure.

One cannot do everything by herself, especially if she's running her own business. Many mothers feel guilty and many just lose their steam trying to keep up, but I know my limitations, and I don't want to kill myself trying to do it all. If people are willing to help or you can afford to hire people to help you, then by all means, take the pressure off of yourself; *get help*, find and surround yourself with a village that will allow you to be the best you. There is nothing wrong with that and nothing wrong with paying someone to help you out.

My village at work is my top team members that can run the office when I'm not present. I rely on my team to make great decisions, and I empower them to do what is needed to make the office the best.

It's important to treat your village with love and respect; after all, they are taking care of you and your family and business. Does the team just come out of nowhere? No, you build trust and you build a team that will respect you and respect the mission of what you are set out to accomplish. There are many careers out there that don't really need a team, but in dentistry, you need several people in order to build your business. Just like a village at home, a village at work is absolutely necessary. The trust you build with your assistants and team members must be a solid and reciprocated relationship. Yes, you pay them, and no, you cannot be their best friend; you are the *boss*. Your team looks to you, as the boss for leadership, but what they want to see most is consistency and stability in you as a leader. If your actions and communication are completely different from what you preach and expect of them, how can you expect your team to be there for you? One of the worst stories I have heard is when a doctor is on maternity leave and she receives a call from her team member stating that she is going to leave for a better offer. When I hear something like that, I am sad for both parties. What does it take to keep your team, and do you do what it takes to keep them? Do you show your appreciation for your team members? Many of you will say, "Yes, of course!" But more often than not, the other person does not feel that way. Sure, there is an exception, a one-off, and perhaps you do have an entitled team member who just demands the world, but for the most part, if you invest enough time and energy into hiring the right person, then treating that person like family—and I mean with respect—will do wonders.

If you ask assistants, why do you stay and why do you like the doctor and or office you work for, what do you think is the most common answer?

My guess is that their boss offers benefits and great pay, that they love the patients, and that they offer great hours; or perhaps they might say, well the doctor is amazing and she really takes care of her team and patients; the doctor respects us as her team and motivates us to do our best and to take pride in our work; the doctor helps us to do our job better and gives us opportunities to grow and learn. What kind of leader do you want to be? What kind of village do you want to have? Ask yourself that and see if you have that or can do better. You are only as good as you can be because you have the right village. Surround yourself with solid people because they are there to help you be the best you can be.

Introducing Dr. Laila Hishaw

In the hilarious and witty book, *Yes Please,* comedian and author, Amy Poehler, exposes the biggest lie many mothers tell themselves: they can do it all alone. She highlights what she refers to as "woman on woman crime," the ongoing finger pointing and judgements on who's raising their children best: stay-at-home or working mothers. The truth is, there are pros and cons to both, but what each have in common is that every

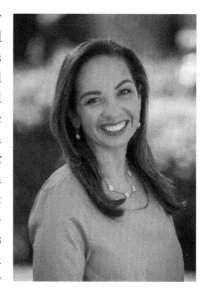

mother needs someone to help her be her best for her family. Amy Poehler's "wife" was her nanny. Maybe yours is your mother, sister, or neighbor. For me, I have more than one person who stands in the gap to nurture my kids when I can't. They step in and help me be the best I can be, so I can be the best for my family. I have a "Village."

It took a village to shape me into who I have become as a wife, a mother, a dentist, a friend, and a successful business woman. My village continues to pour into my family and me so we can live a life of passion, purpose, and happiness. Over the years, the village has changed, manifesting itself in so many ways as I grow. For example, as a young girl raised by a single mother of three, my grandmother lived with us to help my mother. She provided warm, home-cooked meals and checked our homework since my mother worked a second job after teaching all day at her high school. There was also my godmother, a respected physician in our community, who served as a role model for me to work hard and strive for excellence. As my mentor, she provided guidance on my educational path that ultimately led me into a great college and later dental school. When I was older, I played a role in our family's village by helping with my younger sisters. Nine and ten years their senior, I was basically the built-in babysitter. My responsibilities included driving them to and from school, dance class and, of course, the mall. All of this was done to keep our family running smoothly. I never felt as though my mother loved me less because she had to work so hard. In fact, she modeled how to be dedicated to her profession which was making an impact on her students' lives. She sacrificed to make sure my sisters and I could achieve any dream we imagined for ourselves. My mother was smart enough to know that she couldn't do it alone and made the conscious effort to surround us with nurturing adults who wanted the best for us too, but offered other gifts and talents to help us succeed. These experiences and connections have molded me into the highly motivated, compassionate leader, role model, and mentor I am today in my dental practice and community. The love I received from my village has shaped me to become a nurturing mother, devoted wife, and supportive friend.

As a "Mommy Dentist in Business" with three busy pediatric dental practices and three amazing, on-the-go kids, I rely heavily on my village. Unfortunately, it has taken me many years to figure that out. As dentists, we are already wired as high achievers who strive for perfection in our work. We often believe that perfection has to carry over into our personal lives as well. We should be able to get up in the morning, make breakfast for the kids, pack up the baby bag for daycare, drop everyone off, get to work and be of clear mind to perform dental surgery for eight hours, then finish charts at the end of the day. After that, we rush out to pick up the kids from after school care and the baby from the daycare. Don't forget about swim practice, dance class, or basketball. Finally, we're home, and it's time to get dinner going, clean up the kitchen, sign reading logs and review spelling words, bathe the kids, read to them, and tuck them in bed. Now it's "me-time" to check emails, RSVP for birthday parties, buy a gift on Amazon, and set a reminder to schedule the kids' doctor's appointment tomorrow at lunch. Have you asked your husband how his day was yet? Oh, and did you try to work out or meditate or do anything for yourself in that craziness? Doesn't it seem insane just to read that? Well, most of us are doing that! Why do we put this pressure on ourselves? Perhaps it's the mommy guilt we carry, but it's time to embrace our inner "Elsa" and LET IT GO! I was killing myself trying to be perfect, and in the end, I was depleted and couldn't give my family what they needed: for me to be truly present in the moment!

It finally clicked when people would say, "I don't know how you do it all!" Well, I wasn't doing it all that well! When I finally recognized that I needed a village just like my mother did, things got better for everyone, including myself. My village has grown to include my nanny, mother, in-laws, sisters, friends, Sunday school teachers, colleagues and my amazing life coach. I realize that not everyone can rely on a loving and reliable partner, but I can…and yet I wasn't. My husband and I got married and started a family together, yet we had fallen into roles and responsibilities that we should have defined better earlier on. Even the most in tune spouses are not mind readers. We are now on the same page about what our children and household require of both of us.

One of the most important things I learned from my life coach, Leslie Fuqua Williams of LFW Coach, is that when I am in the whirlwind of the busyness and stressfulness of my day, I can't allow it to blur my focus on what my values are. Focusing on my values will keep me aligned with my moral principles which are faith, family, friends, and community. I have integral people in each of those areas that make up my village, but I want to share with you why I value the relationships in my communities and how they impact my life.

Mommy Dentists in Business is a community that brings together mothers from around the globe that share two common interests: being a mom and a dentist. We share unique experiences that no one else would appreciate or understand. I have gained knowledge, support, inspiration, and friendships from this group that has helped me improve my practice and my soul. It has also given me the grace to forgive myself when I feel I have fallen short of being a super mom! Thank you, Dr. Grace Yum, for creating and protecting this community for us!

I've made sure to involve myself with communities that nurture my children too. All mothers want their children to be strong in their confidence and self-esteem, and sometimes that is affected by whom they are surrounded. For African American children, this is especially important, which I recently witnessed with my teenage daughter. After being at a conference and seeing other girls who look like her embracing who they were, she was inspired to do the same. She is proud of who she is and no longer feels like she must be someone else to fit in. Having this organization in my village is providing strength to my children through leadership development, volunteer service, philanthropic giving, and civic duty. Thank you, Jack and Jill of America, Inc!

My circle of friends makes up another community in my village. Most Saturdays, my husband and I engage in our "Divide & Conquer" mode when all three kids must be at three different places. We often need to call on a friend to help us, and they are always there. Sometimes your friend will be the one to save your life. This was the case when my physician friend encouraged me to get a mammogram after I turned 40 years old. I pushed back that I wasn't a high risk. Thankfully, she continued to persist, and we were able to catch my breast cancer at the earliest stages. I write this as I celebrate my 5-year anniversary of being cancer free this month! Cultivating my friendships keeps me both grounded and uplifted. I can trust them to tell me the truth even when it's hard to hear. You know who you are. I love you all!

My village represents a community of people whose relationships have been the key to my success. From that success, it was natural to want to pay it forward and be a member of someone else's village. What we don't realize as Mommy Dentists is that we are so much more than a doctor who fixes teeth and prevents oral disease. We serve as role models and mentors to children and future dentists. It's incumbent on us to nurture and bring up the next generation of leaders in our field. I recently discovered that black dentists make up only 3.8% of all dentists in America. I have always believed that representation matters and that children will want to emulate that which they see in their lives. As a result, I decided something needed to be done to change this statistic. I created the Diversity in Dentistry Mentorship

Facebook Forum to educate and expose young African American youth and other underrepresented minorities to dentistry. I want to share that dentistry is a rewarding career and is an attainable goal early on in life so they are on the right educational path to be successful candidates for dental school and, ultimately, valuable leaders in the profession of dentistry. Oprah has said, "A mentor is someone who allows you to see the hope inside yourself." What greater feeling is there than being that person for someone else?

Writing this chapter has helped me realize just how diverse and impactful my village has been. Honoring everyone in it has given me an indescribable sense of gratitude. My village has been, and continues to be, the key to my success. Have you tapped into your village lately? You are not in this world alone! Reach out and embrace the help offered by others who cares for you and your family so you can live the life you deserve. Mommy Dentists in Business can do it all. It just takes a village!

Dr. Laila Hishaw is a private practice pediatric dentist and owner at Tucson Smiles Pediatric Dentistry in Tucson, Arizona and Diplomate of the American Board of Pediatric Dentistry. Her compassionate nature with her colleagues and patients has brought her recognition as one of Tucson's Top Dentist™ and featured on "Mystery Diagnosis" on Discovery Health Channel. As a mother of three and an owner of three practices, work/life balance has been the proverbial challenge. Dr. Hishaw is sharing the lessons she learned to create balance by acknowledging the power of her village, who reminds her she is not alone. To connect with Dr. Hishaw, please visit www.DrLailaHishaw.com.

Chapter Fourteen
What is Your WHY?

What is your WHY is a question that I both love and hate at the same time because I'm afraid of my answer...I think. This question has become such a catch phrase among consultants and coaches that it seems cliché, but if you really sit down and think about it, I think there is a good lesson in going through the process; the answer to the question may change from time to time because the season of whatever it is you are going through can change. When I reflect on my why right now in this instance, it definitely isn't the same as last year. My why has evolved into something bigger and greater than me and it just seems that things have fallen into my lap, as if the universe is handing me something and I need to figure out what to do with it.

Up until now, my why has been very clear: be a pediatric dentist, treat patients because you care about them and want them to have great health, own your own business so that you can be your own boss, be an amazing wife and mom. But now in my 40's, I'm experiencing this shift and it's uncomfortable. Why is it uncomfortable? It is because for the first time in my life I'm not exactly sure what I'm supposed to do. I have reached the pinnacle in my career and I'm finding out that I can either keep things the way they are and continue on in my practice or I can make a change in my career. I can still practice, but now I can move in a different direction. I think that many people come to this point in their careers where they question what is next. Should I become a speaker? Should I become a dental consultant? Should I just retire? No, I could not retire now…actually being a stay at home mom would drive me crazy. I've concluded that I should just let things take their course. To accept opportunities where they may lie and see where things take me. This is the exact opposite philosophy from what I grew up with and goes against every grain in my body. Yet, I am going to embrace the present and enjoy my journey!

You see, I'm the person that likes to plan everything out way in advance. I usually have a clear-cut path in my goals and in my life. People ask me all the time, "Why do you feel the need to be a business owner? Why do you need to own two dental offices? Why do you need to work full time if your husband is able to support your family? Why do you have to work so much?" It's because I am an overachiever, and I don't ever want to stop! I like that feeling of being driven and feeling like I have accomplished achievements beyond what my colleagues are doing. It's not a competitive thing; it is more that I have a desire for achievement. I guess you can call me an overachiever. It's just part of who I am ever since I was a child. I grew up with a "tiger dad" and sometimes "tiger mom" and if I brought home less than an A, they reprimanded me. That drove me into becoming a perfectionist and always wanting to have a plan! I'm the person who always knows where I am going and what I'm doing. I even planned out when my first and second child needed to be born. My husband and I were at a Chinese restaurant with white paper on the table. I wrote down all the months and counted the number of months backwards from December to plan my pregnancy. That is how crazy I am! I even researched how to conceive a girl versus a boy…and got my son.

Sometimes it's almost easier not to think about what your "why" is because it feels daunting. No matter what I do, I feel that maybe it's not enough. The way I combat that is basically not to think too much about it or not think too deeply. My thoughts are just to do my best and the best will have to be good enough! It took me a long time to get here, and to think about all the things I could be doing better just drained all my energy. So rather than focusing on the trivial things that bog me down, I would prefer to focus on the things that really matter to me in the big picture. I want my children to be proud of their mom. I want them to see that moms can have careers and be with their children too. I want my kids to see that their mother works hard to provide for them and send them a message that mommy can be an independent professional and that they too can achieve whatever it is they want to if they work hard! I want them to see that hard work can bring success.

I also love that my husband is so supportive of me and that he knows that I can handle business situations on my own, that if something were to happen to him we will be okay.

The "BIG WHY", as in why I am a pediatric dentist, is that this is my calling. I truly believe that the Lord has called me into this profession to help children and families. I believe that ever since I was in college working in dental offices and meeting the doctors, they mentored me and paved a path to be where I am now. I believe that doors open for a reason and God closes doors when needed. My whole life has been centered around what the Lord has provided for me, given that I have worked hard for it. My path was pretty certain and it was never easy, but I worked hard! I was never the genius child, I was always the one that needed to try really hard and put in 110% effort. Nothing was ever easy!

But fast forward to today. God is changing my direction once again. Back in June of 2017, I started Mommy Dentists in Business Facebook Group in New Orleans, sitting in the Roosevelt Hotel at a law firm gala with my husband. I was waiting for him to be done so that we could go home, and out of half boredom and half motivation, I started the group. I thought, if lawyers can get together and share information, why can't dentists? I had been in some of the dental groups before, but I wanted something more specific. I wanted something more for myself and connect with other moms that were doing what I was doing, which is raising kids and running a business! The birthplace of MDIBS was in New Orleans. As we were on our way to the airport headed home, people were joining every hour. My phone kept on receiving notifications that more and more people were joining. I initially added my friends from school and thought that it would just be them. But it kept growing and growing, and we are over 4,000 members and global! My "why" has evolved this year because of this group. At first, it was just to have comradery, but now my "why" has changed to helping other mom dentists to be the best that they can be and to encourage them to keep on keeping on!

Introducing Dr. Alisa Nelson-Wade

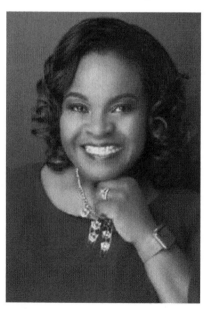

My journey is not really unlike most of yours. At first, we are kids having kid experiences. The next thing we know...Bam! We are adults leading adult lives. Husbands, kids, practices, patients, employers, employees, extended family, and friends are all the things to which we dedicate our lives (both personal and professional). They are also the things that we tend to lose our "self" too. We become so immersed in the daily task of taking care of all the needs of the ones that are essential to our lives and livelihood; we forget the person we once stared face to face in the mirror and promised to always be there for; before anything or anyone else.

At some point in our busy lives and fruitful careers as Mommy Dentists, we may find ourselves sitting back and taking an aerial assessment of our existence and ask the question, "Why?". If you are like me and have a strong, first-name-basis relationship with Jesus; you'd be a little more specific and ask "Jesus, why am I here and why is my life this way?" Now, if you have an unabashed sense of boldness you may have the audacity to ask, "What is my purpose?"

I cannot only remember the day that I asked God these very questions (unabashed boldness included), but I also remember the very day he answered. I call this time in my life "My Absolute Epiphany". I had an undoubtedly sudden realization that changed my life.

As usual, I had taken on way more commitments than my schedule, life, physical, and mental abilities could manage. The upcoming weekend, I would be attending a women's conference chalk full of late-night mixers, days of breakout sessions and panel discussion of which I was a major contributor. This meant I had to spend weeks ahead of the actual event researching topics, preparing notes, and organizing thoughts. My husband, a full-time cop, was back and forth in training for a new position. This left me home alone with the kids serving as mom, dad, and chauffeur in addition to being in the midst of preparation. My plate was really full to say the least. Let us not forget that I was still working all day every day in a practice that I swear should have its own reality show.

By mid-week, I hit a wall. My mind was reeling. I was exhausted beyond measure, and I felt no one noticed my state of mind at all. I just sat in my office, closed my eyes, and whispered,

"God, why am I here? It ain't supposed to be like this. I didn't ask for this at all! Why Lord, why?"

As soon as the thought completed itself in my mind, just like clock-work; my office manager knocked on my door asking if we could fit in one more patient. It was the mother of two kids that were already scheduled. Now since they were Medicaid and we had already met the Medicaid patient allowance for this time slot, my answer would have normally been "no". I guess I had reached that street I like to call "whitt's end" but at this point it did not matter.

I told my office manager to add her in and I would take a look. I made my way to the clinic floor. Neck throbbing with the tension of the week, head pounding from lack of sleep and maybe even a little dehydration (I don't like to drink too much water at work as peeing would just slow my daily productivity...please say I'm not the only one of us who avoids drinking liquids at work for this reason).

I saw the mom sitting in the chair being examined by the hygienist. She noticed me and took a break from the conversation to do the introduction and give me the patient's back story. I eek out a half-smile and introduce myself; mustering up enough energy so that my body language says, "I am so glad to see you."

So wrapped up in my own stuff, I robotically reach for the patient's chart information and give it a once over. I quickly glanced her way and immediately notice something about her eyes that gave me pause. I can still remember that look today. Her eyes were a sad, empty, dark window to what I would soon find out gave view to a desperate soul.

At that moment, the tension in my neck and the pounding in my head faded into the sadness I saw in these beautifully hazel yet pensive eyes. Even the full bladder was no match for the lump forming in my throat as I felt the Holy Spirit take control of my lips to ask her what brought her in to see me today.

She said to me, "Thank you for seeing me and my kids today, Dr. Nelson. You and your staff have always been nice to my children so I wanted to get my teeth cleaned. I do not have anything. My husband left me and the kids with nothing. I can barely take care of them. I can't find a job and I stay in constant pain. I had planned to bring them here, get them something to eat and then go home tonight and kill myself."

My heart stopped and the room began to move in slow motion as she spoke to me. I looked into those eyes that told me so much as tears began to form in their corners; making little streams down her cheeks.

From this point, I don't remember anything but clearing that treatment room, sitting up her chair, and grabbing her hand. The Holy Spirit did what it so amazingly does. I stayed there with her until we had a therapist on the phone who could see her immediately. My staff and I made sure that she got to therapy. We also made sure her kids (our babies) were okay as well.

Later that day as I sat in that same office chair that I had complained to God about my life; I heard him say to me so clearly, "Lisa this is your why! Dentistry is your Ministry. I allow you to be here to do dentistry, sure, but your main purpose is to show your patients and the world my unconditional love. To let them know who I am and how much I love them. You can do that here with no hindrance or reservation. As long as you do, you will never want for anything."

I could not contain myself. I began to sob uncontrollably. I cry even now just thinking about it. It has never been about me, my wants, or my needs. God has elevated me and all of us to these positions for a purpose...His Purpose.

I realized my why, my purpose, is to glorify him and show the world what true love (Agape love) really is. I don't complain (as much) any more. I don't have to overextend myself anymore either. I realize now that this was just a defense mechanism I used to cope with being unsure of who I was in this life and profession.

I challenge each of you mommies to ask yourselves these questions. "What is my WHY? What is my purpose?"

I can almost guarantee it is a lot bigger than "spinning" and handpiece! God Bless you all and I can't wait to see you all on this side of "Why"!

Dr. Alisa Nelson-Wade received her Doctorate of Dental Surgery (DDS) from Meharry Medical College. After residency training, she was invited to serve as an Associate Professor in the department of Periodontics and Oral Diagnosis, eventually rising to Clinical Course Coordinator.

Desiring a more fast-paced environment, Dr. Nelson-Wade moved back to Georgia to try her hand in corporate dentistry. She quickly found that she desired more personal relationships with her patients, leading to her opening Comfort Dental Studio, P.C. which quickly grew out of its store-front location. She then relocated the practice to Grayson, Georgia; making her the first African American to own Commercial property in the city of Grayson.

A native of Eatonton, Georgia, Dr. Alisa has shared her message of perseverance in churches, classrooms and seminars since 1999. Her recently published book: **"Imitating the Tree: The Journey to Your Purpose and Destiny"** (a dramatic, spiritual narrative about her struggles with life, love, and family) has received rave reviews all across the country. Dr. Alisa also serves as Minister at Hopewell Northeast Baptist Church where she is under the leadership of Senior Pastor Gerard Blanding, Sr and Co-Pastor Veta Blanding.

In addition to being a respected dentist, entrepreneur and author, over the course of her career, Dr. Alisa has received many honors and awards. She has been a member of many dental and civic organizations; including the American Dental Association, the Academy of General Dentistry, The National Dental Association and of course Delta Sigma Theta Sorority, Inc. She is the doting wife of Mr. Lawrence Wade and proud mother to Nicholas and Natalie.

Dr. Alisa Nelson-Wade is currently available as a keynote speaker for inspirational events, as well as business organizations, churches and community events. For more information or media inquiries please contact Alisa at anelson0128@gmail.com.

Chapter Fifteen
Your Health is Everything

For as long as I can remember, I've struggled with my health. I was always overweight and have never had the best body image. It started when I was probably around 10 years old. Maybe it was right before puberty that I put on a lot of weight. My pediatrician always told me that I was at least 10 pounds overweight and that I needed to lose weight. I was also made fun of by my family members, i.e. aunts, uncles, and cousins. My sister, on the other hand, was tall and skinny; I was short and fat. My classmates at school made fun of me as well. In junior high, I clearly remember an incident in the lunch room when I wanted to sit next to my friend Sara. There was a boy sitting next to her and when I came over, he told me that there wasn't enough room for me because I was too fat. Of course, tears were swelling up in me and I froze because I didn't know what to do. Luckily, my friends came to my side, buzzed him off, and made arrangements for me, but those painful incidents never subsided and came up repeatedly. This, of course, carried over into high school, and along with the extra weight came the pimples and braces. That was a super atrocious time for me because I just never wanted to go anywhere.

One day, my freshman year, I remember my mother forced me to take up a sport because she heard that colleges look for team sports participation. She took me over to the swim team and talked to the coach. He asked if I knew how to swim, and of course, I said yes, I knew how to swim. What I didn't know was that he meant how to swim like a professional and not just be wading around and playing diving games in the pool. That was my first experience in being a part of something other than the orchestra. I was an excellent violinist, but a horrendous athlete. My sister, Anna, on the other hand, was a complete superstar and excelled at anything she did; she tested into the gifted and talented program at my school; she was the captain of her basketball and track/field team; she won state championship when she was on the basketball team; she even played the cello and brought home great grades. Then there was me: overweight, not that great at sports, but I did well at the violin and at school. I was a straight-A student until high school.

Joining the swim team was turned out to be a great idea. My weight was finally under control, and for the first time, I felt really confident in myself. I was a part of a team and I became a pretty decent swimmer, minus the butterfly stroke; I was more like the drowning butterfly. My sister, of course, helped boost my confidence. She is a natural athlete and just amazing at any sport she wants to pick up. Take her golfing and she will swing a club like a professional. While I was a swimmer, she became a diver, which was way cooler than being a swimmer, but it was fun to do those things with her.

As I got older and went on to college at Northwestern, I gained the typical freshman 15. I remember when my father picked me up from school to go home for the summer. It was funny how he commented on how terrible I looked. I can always rely on my parents to be completely honest with me. Needless to say, the freshman 15 never really went away until I went to dental school. I remember being extremely self-conscious and always had people commenting on my weight. But when I went to dental school, something just happened. I don't know exactly why, but the weight just started coming off. I attribute it to not having time to go out to eat and having a grueling schedule. But when I returned home from dental school everyone was so surprised at the weight loss. I felt better and looked better! I started to work out more and really watched my diet.

Now in my 40's I try hard to squeeze in exercise about two times a week. I love to practice yoga as it helps to stretch me out and work on areas that feel tight due to my work as a dentist. Most dentists are tight in the neck, shoulder, back area so it is always a great idea to stretch and get massages regularly to stay fit and healthy! If you want to practice a long time, it is important to take care of your body!

An Interview with Dr. Teresa Scott

1. When did you feel your health was in jeopardy?

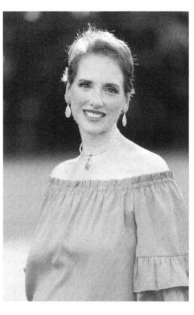

My health has been crappy my whole life, so I have never really had good health, which means my descent into jeopardy was a slow, steady decline; over decades. Had I known then what I know now! I started out with six sets of tubes in my ears as a young child; multiple bouts of bronchitis and reactive airway issues. When I was 16 years old, I had my first ovarian cyst; it was the size of a large melon, and it was removed, after which my period stopped completely and I gained 100 pounds in a single year—my freshman year of college. I had more bronchitis and reactive airway issues, then my second ovarian cyst at 26; this one ruptured but I didn't have surgery. The third one was at age 31; that one was the size of a grapefruit; I was septic and needed IV antibiotics for six weeks. It was also the first time someone actually finally diagnosed me with polycystic ovarian syndrome.

I couldn't get anyone to listen to my complaints; they all just thought I was fat and lazy and addicted to food because I was also 390 pounds by that point. I tried every single diet out there, and none of them worked. And it wasn't because I was cheating, because I wasn't. Anyway, four months later, I ended up with a hernia the size of a football—all my internal sutures had ripped. The doctors fixed my hernia, but 18 months later, the hernia repair gave way and I ended up with a bowel obstruction. *That* was traumatic, because my intestines reversed and went the opposite direction. *Totally* reversed. You can imagine what is coming out of your mouth...BLECH! I asked the doctor why this kept happening to me, and he said that it was because of my weight. I told him, "What part of Polycystic Ovarian Syndrome do you not understand?! I *can't* lose weight." He recommended that I get a gastric bypass and that it would reset my metabolism.

It took me about nine months, but I finally convinced the insurance company to pay for the surgery. I lost 222 pounds in 18 months and my weight has stayed relatively stable since then. My metabolism reset itself. Sounds great right? Ah...had I known then what I know now. I got my period back after 20 years of infertility. I ended up pregnant with my oldest at age 37, and she was a total surprise. I gave birth to her at age 38. The pregnancy was unremarkable; easy, in fact. I thought I was finally free from health issues. I had a c-section, like many women seem to nowadays, so I thought nothing of it. I ended up with another hernia where my c-section had been. Apparently, I herniate easily!

Nine months after my first was born, I became pregnant with my youngest. My second pregnancy was a harder one. She was very active, and she kicked me so hard that she turned the hernia that *was* six inches long into a 12-inch-long rip. It went from my hip bone to my diaphragm towards the end of my 32nd week. Every time she moved, the hernia ripped a little bit more. I was bleeding from it slowly. They admitted me into the hospital at 32 weeks, and my blood tests showed that I was missing half of my blood, but nobody could figure out why. The only thing normal about my blood was my platelets, and honestly, if I was missing half of my blood, I should have been missing half of my platelets too.

Apparently, the doctor didn't read the previous OB's genetic testing that showed a Leiden Factor V deficiency, making me vulnerable to Deep Vein Thrombosis (DVTs). Anyway, I ended up with a DVT at 32 weeks 4 days, so they did an emergency filter basket placement the next day, and the day after that, my youngest was born at 32 weeks 6 days. The doctor told me that my insides looked like a starving victim from Somalia. I didn't really *get* what that meant, other than I was missing half my blood, and the rip in my side explained that. Anyway, the baby was in the NICU for three-and-a-half weeks but did fine. I was back at work with an emergency patient four days later, because I felt fine now that my insides were not being ripped every time she moved. It's important to know this, because it speaks to how I recover from surgeries; I'm up and walking within 12 hours, and I am usually off of pain meds that are stronger than Advil within four days.

After she was born, I ended up with a litany of complaints—my joints hurt, I had full body cramps, my intestines were always irritated. I put on weight even though I was not eating badly (compared to the standard American diet). Around the time my youngest was born, I was introduced to holistic approaches to medicine, so I was into essential oils and eating healthy and raw milk—all things my children were totally thriving on—and yet my own health continued to decline. When my oldest was 5 years old, we went gluten free as a family (she ended up with a gluten and dairy intolerance after vaccinations. I put that together later). My oldest child had ADD issues and her kindergarten teachers were starting to make noises about Ritalin. I was damned if I was going to let my child hop on the pharmaceutical train that had become my life. I was on 12 different prescriptions at that point.

Going gluten free helped tremendously. My joint pain stopped. My muscle cramping, my constipation/diarrhea cycles, my thyroid normalized. I lost 35 pounds without doing anything else other than eliminating gluten from my diet. Again, I felt like I was on an upswing. I was able to lose nine of the prescriptions, but the sleeping part was getting worse and worse. Towards the end of 2014, I was getting maybe two-and-a-half hours of sleep per night. It was a nightmare. I spent my weekend days in bed, trying to sleep because I had not gotten any real sleep during the week. I abandoned my children to my husband's care to try to get some sleep. I probably was close to psychotic by the end of 2014. I was *desperate*, in a way that nobody should ever have to be. Whenever I went to regular MDs, they would prescribe me sleeping pills or antidepressants (but I wasn't depressed), which didn't work. I didn't really develop a habit (because from what I have heard, Xanax and other benzodiazepines are really hard to kick once you are on them), but I did convince myself I needed more of them because they didn't work for me as well as for other people.

I thought it was because of the gastric bypass—that I wasn't absorbing the medicine.

I saw a holistic MD on February 2, 2015. She recognized my symptoms as malnutrition and systemic candidiasis and perimenopause. She put me on two antifungals and a regimen of bioidentical hormones and nutritional supplements. I stopped the sleeping pills cold turkey because they clearly weren't the answer anyway. Thank God I didn't have a true dependence on them, because otherwise, I would have gone through some serious withdrawals. I went through none. Six days later, I was finally sleeping on my own for longer than two-and-a-half hours per night. Within three weeks, I was getting a full seven hours of sleep a night. It was a miracle. I spent some time recovering. For the next few months, I felt pretty good for the first time *ever*, but my periods started acting weird. I started getting this discharge that was clear, serosanguinous liquid, and it was not my period. I figured it was the bioidentical hormones helping my body regulate, so I didn't think too much of it, but by August of 2015, I was filling a pad each day with that discharge, so I made an appointment with the gynecologist.

It took six weeks to be seen, so they saw me at the end of September 2015, and did a PAP smear. It came back clean, so they brought me back to do an ultrasound. The doctor found a thickening of the uterus during the ultrasound as well as another ovarian cyst, and she said that the thickening of the uterus was concerning to her. She did a biopsy and that same day, my hip started to hurt; it was nagging. I thought it was my hernia, which was the size of a basketball by that time, but Advil had been enough for me. She called me back October 7, 2015 and said it was cancer and we needed to make an appointment with a gynecological oncologist because I needed to get a hysterectomy. She thought it would be fine because the lesion was small and didn't look like it had gone through the wall of the endometrium. It looked like stage I cancer, so we scheduled the surgery for October 29, 2015.

Within those three weeks, that nagging pain in my hip became stronger and almost constant. And then it became intractable. Advil and Tylenol did nothing to help by the night before the surgery came, so I checked into the emergency room in tears, telling them that the surgery was scheduled for the next day, but that the pain was horrible and I didn't know what else to do. Something most people don't know about me—I don't respond to medications. At. All. It should have been a clue to me as to why the sleeping pills the doctors prescribed didn't feel like they did anything. It's because they didn't. Prescription narcotics don't affect me either. This is a harbinger of what was to come.

Anyway, bright and early the next morning, they took me into surgery. I informed them that pain management is problematic for me, and requested that they do an epidural for pain control, since narcotics don't work for me. They humored me, but fully intended to give me narcotics anyway. Hospital personnel never listen to me. It usually takes 36 hours of pain after any surgery for them to listen; this time, it took 56 hours. I guess they were denser than usual. I requested Toradol and Tramadol—the only two things that have worked in the past; they worked beautifully after my c-sections. I woke up from surgery in horrific pain. It was at least a 15 on a scale of 1-10. Over the next 56 hours, I begged to die. They finally did the epidural. I couldn't feel my feet, but I could surely feel the pain in my hip. Nothing they gave me worked. Morphine, Dilaudid, Fentanyl, Oxycontin, Demerol, IV Tylenol. They finally gave in and gave me the Toradol and the tramadol. To my horror, *nothing* worked, so for the first 56 hours after surgery, I truly did beg to die. I asked them to put me in a coma; they refused. The post-operative pain started getting a bit better after 72 hours, so they let me go home, but the hip pain actually increased. They told me it was post-op pain.

Remember, I am the lady that saw an emergency patient four days after my last c-section and didn't need pain medications by then. I am a tough cookie. It takes a *lot* to make me complain, so the pain had to be pretty darn bad for me, and everyone just kept saying it was post-op pain. I have been through a total of 13 abdominal surgeries. I *promise* that I know what post-op pain feels like. This was far worse. Anyway, I went to the oncologist for my two weeks post op, and he told me I was healing well and that the lymph nodes had all come back clean, so no more cancer, right? I was so grateful, but still in horrible pain. I went to a pain management doctor towards the end of November, and he thought it was some ligament that was stretched and pulling my psoas muscle in my back, and several other such nonsense things that he attributed to post-op pain.

He did a procedure where he injected my lower back with some kind of anesthetic and a steroid. It did nothing. I limped away from that appointment in just as much pain, but my lower back was numb. It didn't do a darn thing for the pain in my hip. I went to the radiation oncologist December 1, 2015. I limped in, dragging my left leg. At that point, I was on a rotating regimen of Advil, Tylenol, Toradol and Tramadol. I was taking something every four hours, and I was scared that my liver and kidneys weren't going to recover from that much medicine. Nothing was working, but if I didn't take the pain medicine, it was bad enough to make me cry. The pain was constantly at a 10 or worse. The meds took it down to an 8, which was not pain free, but it was better than a 10.

The radiation oncologist asked me why I was limping. I told her the saga of my pain. She said "well, I need to do a CT scan to measure you for your brachytherapy, but I can widen the scope of the scan to see what is going on in that area." It was supposed to just be radiation around the stump of the cervix. 15 minutes later, I had my answer. She found the metastasis in my anterior superior iliac crest. She asked when my last CT scan was. I said "October 29—just five weeks ago." She accessed the hospital records of the CT scan from October 29th. She found the metastasis on that CT scan. The other doctors had missed it. She compared the lesion to the one from December 1. The lesion had *quadrupled* in size in five weeks. That explained my intractable pain. Bone cancer pain is the worst kind of pain a human being has ever had to feel.

Try to imagine someone has a branding iron red hot in the fire, they stab it into your hip bone, and then they root around for jollies. *That* is what it felt like, so at that point she said that the brachytherapy was a moot point because it was supposed to prevent the spread of metastases and my cancer had already metastasized. She said that at that point, radiation was only going to be effective for palliative measures. Because none of the pharmaceuticals work for me, the radiation would take away the pain for me. She scheduled a confirmation biopsy for December 4, and we started the first of 13 radiation sessions on December 7. I only agreed to the radiation due to desperation about my pain. I would not have done it otherwise.

I already knew that I did not want to do chemo. Every person I knew of who had gone through chemo had died and they were miserable in the process. I asked the question: what is the prognosis? You know the doctor is unwilling to be straight with you when their answer is something like, "It's not curable, but it's treatable," and "Well, nobody can really say how long anyone has, right?" And, "we can make you comfortable." They all lie. They don't know how to be straight with someone because if they are actually straight with them, a lot of people will choose to go home and die. Some might even kill themselves. They try to couch everything in euphemisms and lies. At this point in my life, I don't even have a shred of trust left for allopathic medicine doctors. *At this point in my life, I think they are all idiots.* Clearly, that is the PTSD talking, but the emotion is very real. I haven't in my entire life met an allopathic doctor who hasn't harmed me. Some are nicer than others; some I love as fantastic human beings, but they have *all* harmed me.

The Hippocratic oath is so far out the window for medicine in America now. Seriously, so I did my own research. Turns out that the five-year survival for grade four, stage IV-b endometrial cancer is 1%, but that the average survival is less than a year *with* chemo. These statistics gave me *no* chance of survival without chemo. Those were the odds I was facing, but I didn't choose to go home and die. I *did* choose to *not* do chemo, however. They tried to scare me about it. They said that I would die sooner. I told them that I was going to die anyway, with a 1% chance of survival, so if that was the case, it would be on *my* terms. I *did* plan the terms of my death. I *did* plan to kill myself. I wasn't depressed. I simply made the choice that if this intractable pain wasn't going to end, I was going to end it myself, because it was unacceptable to me to live in that state, and it was unacceptable to me to have my family watch me suffer with their hands tied behind their backs, unable to do a thing to help me or alleviate my pain.

It's cruel and inhuman what the allopathic world does to human beings. They *say* they are helping us. They *lie.* They are not helping us. They are not interested in truly healing us. They are interested in making people dependent before they finally just die. They have *no* interest in actually helping us heal, because sick people are a cash cow. Healthy people don't make them any money. Chemo would have taken away my hands, my brain, my eyes, and my ears, and eventually, it would have killed me; those are all side effects of the chemo they wanted to use. I would have been dead before I actually died. No thanks, so I made my own rules. While I was going through the radiation treatments, I researched holistic cancer treatment centers. Here is a hint about what I learned. Don't go to the cheapest one you can find, but the expensive ones may not work for you either. You may not need to go to one at all if you find the right functional medicine practitioner. Do your research. Figure out if it's something you can work with a good naturopath on, or if you really need a treatment that isn't available in the US—because some truly helpful things are banned here. Seriously.

2. What did you feel when you were facing your doctor and he or she told you of your cancer diagnosis?

I felt shock, of course. Then it was the whole trying-to-process-it thing. Then I was pissed off at God. Then I was determined to fight. I felt sorry for myself for a little while. My personality doesn't really allow me to wallow in self-pity. I take stock of where I am, allow myself a brief period of wallowing, analyze it, and then move forward, because looking back, blaming anyone, etc., is simply not productive. I would rather focus on what I can do to improve things moving forward.

3. What did you do after you found out?

I cried. I went and took a shower, bawled my eyes out for about a good half hour. And then I dried myself off, picked myself up, and made plans for what to do. I started a *ton* of research to try to find answers. I was shooting in every direction, without aiming in any particular one, because I didn't know enough about how to fight this beast to know what to shoot at first.

4. In what way do you think dentists or other career-focused women should take better care of themselves?

Well, honestly, the most important thing is nutrition. I healed myself with nutrition, and I have to fight harder than anyone else, because I have a short gut due to gastric bypass. If I can do it with crappy absorption, anyone can do this, but it's not *just* nutrition; it's a combination of things. It's stress management, nutritional management, hormone management, exercise, and proper detoxification. Dentists in particular are vulnerable to toxins. Most allopathic dentists think people like me are crazy for wearing the space suit when we remove amalgams, but mercury is toxic. A study just came out by the CDC that shows that dentists are something like 23 *times* more likely to get pulmonary fibrosis than the average person is—even accounting for other jobs that are also toxic, right? And yet, the ADA and all our governing bodies tell us that our profession is perfectly safe. *They lie to us*, because if they told us the truth, nobody would be willing to spend a half million dollars of student loans (which is what it sits at about now) to go in to a job that is going to cause them harm. I'm beginning to think we need to wear the space suit *more* than for just amalgam removals.

5. How did it affect your practice as you were going through this journey?

Well, I'm the sole provider for my family. If I don't work, we don't get paid, so we went from being relatively debt free (other than my practice loan and my house mortgage) to being deeply in debt. Again. Holistic cancer treatment isn't cheap! We are still trying to climb out of the abyss. It's slow going. I'm not sure I'm ever going to be financially secure. My team members are superb now. It didn't used to be that way. On this journey, I have learned to be a better leader. I was a toxic leader years ago; codependent, and truthfully, a mess. My health was a mess. My leadership skills were a mess. I was a hot mess, but *everything* in my life has grown for the better. I am a better person now. I am a decent leader. I have learned how to be a transformational leader, instead of a transactional one. That has been powerful.

My team members stuck by me in my hour of need. I actually hired a couple of them in the midst of my battle because some old ones had left just before my diagnosis. I fully disclosed to them about my health, and they still stuck by me. They made sure to help and they never disclosed my situation to my patients because they didn't want to scare them off. They were worried about me and asked me to do. I explained to them the same things I have explained here. They saw me doing all of this healing by myself *and* working at the same time. They saw me getting better, and they cheered me on. My hygienists saw existing patients for cleanings while I was gone. I took some time off, but not much. Who can afford that? Once I was able to work again, I worked six days a week for months to make up for the time I lost and they never complained, not once. It took me the better part of a year to get my business back on its feet. And surprisingly, it grew! 2016 was a banner year for me, even though I had had to take so much time off. 2017 was even bigger. My business has taken off to the point where I now have a part time associate who comes to work with me a day a week. The goal is to grow him to be my full-time associate and then eventually my partner. One day, maybe we'll take on another partner. I have big plans! I want to create an integrative medical center in the North Houston area. I want to bring together different practitioners, *all* of whom approach integrative medicine with a functional medicine philosophy, who have the chops to prescribe allopathic things when necessary, but who choose to prescribe natural modalities when possible.

6. What would you do differently in your younger age?

If I coulda, shoulda, woulda, I would have learned about natural medicine sooner. I would have fixed my diet *much* sooner. I would have not taken an antibiotic unless I was truly septic, and I would have learned about the importance of the microbiome and what gut health means. I would have learned sooner about the importance of these five areas—nutrition, toxins, stress, hormones, and exercise. I still don't have it down; I learn more every day. Exercise is torture for me, so I'm more sedentary than I'd like. I need a friendly bully; someone to come get me out of my chair and make me move, but not in a way that I hate them for it. I need to stop being afraid of hormones. I'm so damned traumatized by what my hormonally-

driven cancer did to me that I'm afraid to take anything that might possibly cause my hormones to increase in a positive way, so I'm still dealing with PTSD, for sure.

Toxins are big things for a dentist. Like *huge*. Had I known then what I know now, I would have become a biological dentist sooner. I *love* my job. I'm good at it, but it's seriously a huge source of toxins. I would not have vaccinated either myself or my kids. I now know that the toxins contained in vaccines set up those who have MTHFR genetic issues for future health issues. That's why my family is gluten intolerant. That is why they had many ear infections as kids. That's why I went through *six* sets of tubes as a kid. That is the reason for a lot of my kids' stuff. MTHFR is a valid reason for a medical exemption from vaccinations. Seriously. Because those who have MTHFR issues don't detox properly. We can't process and eliminate toxins properly. And no matter what the conventional medical approaches tell you, vaccines are full of toxins. They are called adjuvants and are designed to create an inflammatory response in your body. That is their purpose, but nobody has truly studied adjuvants in and of themselves, minus the diseases they are inoculating for. They have *no* idea what the lifelong and generational epigenetic responses are going to be to their drugs. They don't study them for long enough, but there is enough evidence at this point for me to say *no more* when it comes to my own family.

A study came out recently that showed that a drug given to rats had epigenetic effects three generations after the first generation stopped taking the drug, and then it takes *nine* generations to undo the damage done in the first place. And the diseases they are inoculating against are mostly trivial. They are a fever and a rash, a fever and diarrhea, or a fever and a cough. Yes, there are some diseases that it might be valuable to consider vaccinating for, *but* because of the adjuvants, and because they no longer make those vaccines single vaccines, it's no longer something I want to do. I am no longer willing to expose myself or my children to those diseases when they are carried by adjuvants. My body does better fighting diseases without the aid of toxic adjuvants. Yes, there are some people who will die; that is the reality of every disease. I wish it wasn't so, but many more are permanently injured or die from the system as it is rigged now with all of the adjuvants. Look at the Gardasil vaccine. *So* many kids totally taken out of their lives—permanently disabled, permanently damaged, some even dead—for a vaccine that doesn't even really prevent the cervical cancer it *says* it prevents. They have no proof that it does—*none*—but it causes permanent neurological damage; premature ovarian failure, actual cases of cervical cancer, encephalitis, and many other side effects, up to and including *death*, for previously healthy kids. **Where there is risk, there should always be fully informed consent.** And the medical community doesn't tell you that you can't sue the manufacturers or the doctors if you or your kids are injured or die from their stuff. Without the ability to sue them, they have *zero* incentive to make things safer and more effective. **Where there is risk, there *must* be accountability.** Our medical system has neither accountability nor true informed consent in the arena of vaccinations, so if I coulda, shoulda, woulda, I would have told my young self some serious truths.

7. How did you continue to see patients during your medical appointments, and did you have help during this time?

I took time off between surgery and when I went to Mexico after radiation. I also took time off when I was still unable to walk. Mostly, we scheduled around the appointments. I worked early or late on Saturdays to make up the time. I really didn't have anyone to help me. I didn't feel I could afford or even find a per diem doctor because my patient population is specialized. They come to see *me*; they refuse to accept anyone else. It's a bit frustrating at times because they would rather wait for two months to see me than to see my associate the next day, and my associate is a good biological dentist too! *But*, we survived; it was okay. My team is phenomenal, so we worked around things as much as possible.

8. What advice would you give to those of us that are battling cancer or illnesses?

First, do your own research, and don't let them *scare* you or bully you into doing what they want you to do. Look at *all* the pros and cons, the risks and benefits, and basically make sure you are choosing your own informed consent, if that makes sense. They are not interested in giving you the full picture with their informed consent. They give you the information that will most likely get you to say yes, *not* the unvarnished truth. It's like voting at the polls; when they put a subject up for vote on the ballot, they will word it in such a way that it makes you feel like the worst kind of person if you don't vote yes to their proposition. Like they will say, "Texas should protect the privacy and safety of women and children in spaces such as bathrooms, locker rooms, and showers in all Texas schools and government buildings." Well, of course they should! But they should also protect the privacy and safety of all citizens in all places. If you vote *no* for this, it makes you feel like the worst kind of person because you *know* that to vote yes on this means that they will be trying to enforce discrimination of a certain portion of society. Pay attention to the working of things. Ask yourself who benefits from this if I say yes. Who gets hurt if I yes. Who benefits from this if I say no. Who gets hurt if I say no. If you can't think of anything or anyone, dig deeper. Unfortunately, *everything* in this life has balancing of good and bad. The key is to figure out where your balance point is.

For example, fevers build immune systems. They are actually a good thing. I try to let my kids fight their illnesses with their fevers unless it goes to 104. I don't give a fever reducer anymore until a fever reaches that level because it means their immune system is doing what it's supposed to do, *but* a fever when a tooth is developing can cause a weak spot in that tooth. We are taught that in dental school, so every good thing has a balancing bad thing. Look for the balancing issues in whatever you are dealing with. Try to remain objective because sometimes, like political issues, it can be a hot-button topic that can take away your objectivity. Look at how things are worded. They pay marketing people a *lot* of money to word things specifically to create a desired emotional response. Learn to see past that to the true nuggets of informational gold underneath.

Second, get the GREECE cancer test. It's not a fix, but it will help you get started with natural substances that work best for *your* body and *your* cancer. If I had done this *before* I went to Mexico, I wouldn't have gone to Mexico, because they didn't treat me there with my greatest cancer fighter: vitamin C. I put myself into remission in 90 days with IV vitamin C. For anyone that says that vitamin C doesn't work for healing, they *lie*. Vitamin C saved my life.

Third, get your nutrition reined in. Seriously. Make it unnegotiable. Don't give in to sugar or gluten; they are addictive and inflammatory. Stick to raw dairy if you do dairy or it's also inflammatory. It has amazing probiotic benefits if it's raw. Become alkaline with your food. Alkalinity is *key* to heath. Invest in pH paper. If you are not alkaline, you are sick. Disease cannot live in an alkaline environment. If your body can't maintain alkalinity in a sustained manner, it's sick. Period. You might feel fine, but it will bite you in the butt.

Fourth, eliminate all sources of toxins from your body and environment. Get the amalgams and root canals out of your mouth if you have them. Other people may be able to handle them, but if you are sick like that, you can't. That means get rid of toxic mold if it is around. Don't continue to subject your body to vaccines. You can't handle them if you are already sick. Drink filtered, fluoride-free water. That means change all your soaps, detergents, lotions, toothpastes, and everything else that touches your body, or washes your dishes or clothes, to things that don't have ANY toxicity potential. Check with the EWG for how toxic something is. If it doesn't rate minimal on their scale, don't use it.

Fifth, exercise. Do as I say, not as I do. I struggle with exercise, but consider purchasing a rebounder. Just six minutes a day on a rebounder is valuable for eliminating toxins.

Sixth, get your hormones under control *naturally*, not with pharmaceuticals. There are plenty of herbs and foods that can help you normalize your hormones. There are plenty of dietary practices that help to normalize them too. Do your research; it's out there. For example, Maca root can help normalize hormones. It's totally natural and over the counter.

Seventh, trite as it sounds, learn to manage your stress. It matters. I'm a type-A, workaholic, and overachiever. I have learned to let a *lot* of things go. I have learned to delegate. I have learned to trust other people to do their jobs. I have learned to not micromanage, and my life has gotten busier since this started, so I am having to learn to carve out long weekends for some time off. Figure out what works for *you*. I am at my happiest when I am helping people; when my mind is engaged in solving a problem somehow, so it's not necessarily about working less, as much as it is about making sure you have a healthy working environment. Work with people you like and respect; that kind of thing.

And last, get your blood tested regularly. Work with a naturopath or functional medicine practitioner who isn't interested in seeing your blood levels look normal. You don't want to be normal; you want to be *optimal*. They are very, very different numbers. I'm *normal* for the first time in 30 years, but I'm not yet optimal. I'm determined to get there, though.

9. What advice would you give to those that are healthy?

Practice prevention now! There is a *huge*, intimate, intricate link between oral health and systemic health. There is such a huge link between chronic inflammation, cancer, Alzheimer's, and other diseases, and it's *so* preventable. We can *all* try to eat healthy now so that we are able to live to 120. Seriously. We can *all* check our blood at least once a year and tweak our results with nutrition and a few key supplements. It's not a difficult thing to do. If a person with stage IV cancer can reverse it with nutrition, then all a healthy person has to do to stay healthy is to start the good habits now. Eat a gluten free, sugar free diet. Manage your stressors. Exercise. Make sure your hormones are balanced naturally. Eliminate toxins from your life. Why wait until you get a devastating diagnosis? Survival isn't guaranteed when you get a diagnosis like mine. It's *so* much more of a guarantee if you are healthy to begin with.

An honors graduate of St. Pius X High School and University of St. Thomas, graduating Magna Cum Laude with a Bachelor's degree in Biology, Teresa Scott went on to extend her education, receiving her doctorate from the University of Texas Health Science Center at San Antonio Dental School.

She received both the Jurisprudence Award, and the Award for Excellence in Clinical Dentistry while still in dental school. She is a member in good standing of the American Dental Association, American Academy of General Dentistry, American Academy of Women Dentists, the Texas Dental Association, the Greater Houston Dental Society, the International Academy of Biological and Dental Medicine, the International Academy of Oral Medicine and Toxicology, the Holistic Dental Association and the American Academy for Oral Systemic Health. She's also won Houston's Top Dentists award from H Texas Magazine (2007 – Present) and America's Top Dentists award from Consumer's Research Council of America (2005 – Present).

Dr. Scott is a true family dentist in every sense of the word. She sees very young children and very old seniors. Her niche has developed among patients suffering from dental phobias or previous negative dental experiences. Her favorite patients are the multi-generational families that she has developed relationships with over the years. She will start out seeing the parents or children, and then move on to include the grandparents, great grandparents, aunts, uncles, cousins and friends and coworkers.

Dr. Scott averages 100% in patient satisfaction. She looks forward to building a lasting, lifelong relationship with all her patients. Dr. Scott has been married to her husband Dan, since 1999, and they have two daughters, Grace and Promise.

To connect with Dr. Scott, please contact her at www.HolisticDentalAssociates.com.

Chapter Sixteen
Conclusion

Thank you for taking the time to read this book that has come from a background of various doctors and their journeys. Not one person's journey is exactly the same as mine even though we are all mommy dentists! We share the joy of graduating dental school, the relief of passing our boards, the happiness in our families, the awesomeness of being a boss, and the blood, sweat, and tears of building a practice. We also share the feelings of mom guilt, the struggles of balancing work and life, the grief of dealing with human resources, and the burden of knowing that other people depend on us for paychecks. But at the end of the day, none of us would trade it for the world. The struggle is real; it really is.

But the sweetness of success would not be so sweet if it were not for the struggle. If you want to be a BOSS, or better yet a MOMBOSS, it is doable. You just have to want to do it! Nothing is better than working on your own terms. There is never the perfect moment to start a practice, just like there isn't the perfect moment to have a child. The world is at your fingertips, and no one will hand you anything on a silver platter. You have to make your own magic! Nothing in life that is worthwhile is easy. As the members of my group would say, "Get it, girl"!